NUTRITION
and the
FEMALE
ATHLETE

NUTRITION in EXERCISE and SPORT

Editors, Ira Wolinsky and James F. Hickson, Jr.

Published Titles

Nutrients as Ergogenic Aids for Sports and Exercise
Luke Bucci

Nutrition in Exercise and Sport, 2nd Edition
Ira Wolinsky and James F. Hickson, Jr.

Exercise and Disease
Ronald R. Watson and Marianne Eisinger

Nutrition Applied to Injury Rehabilitation and Sports Medicine
Luke Bucci

Nutrition for the Recreational Athlete
Catherine G.R. Jackson

NUTRITION in EXERCISE and SPORT

Editor, Ira Wolinsky

Published Titles

Nutrition, Physical Activity, and Health in Early Life
Jana Parízková

Exercise and Immune Function
Laurie Hoffman-Goetz

Sports Nutrition: Minerals and Electrolytes
Constance Kies and Judy Driskell

Nutrition and the Female Athlete
Jaime S. Ruud

Body Fluid Balance: Exercise and Sport
E.R. Buskirk and S. Puhl

Forthcoming Titles

Biochemical Methods for Exercise Assessment
Jon Karl Linderman
Sports Nutrition: Vitamins and Trace Elements
Ira Wolinsky and Judy Driskell

Amino Acids and Proteins for the Athlete — The Anabolic Edge
Mauro G. Pasquale

NUTRITION
and the
FEMALE
ATHLETE

Jaime S. Ruud, M.S., R.D.

Nutrition Consultant
Lincoln, Nebraska

CRC Press
Boca Raton   New York   London   Tokyo

Library of Congress Cataloging-in-Publication Data

Ruud, Jaime S.
    Nutrition and the female athlete / Jaime S. Ruud.
        p. cm.
    Includes bibliographical references and index.
    ISBN 0-8493-7917-2 (alk. paper)
    1. Athletes--Nutrition. 2. Women--Nutrition. I. Title.
TX361.A8R88   1996
613.2′ 024796--dc20   96-11966
                                                           CIP

No claim to original U.S. Government works
International Standard Book Number 0-8493-7917-2
Library of Congress Card Number 96-11966
Printed in the United States of America 1 2 3 4 5 6 7 8 9 0
Printed on acid-free paper

SERIES PREFACE

The CRC series on Nutrition in Exercise and Sport provides a setting for in-depth exploration of the many and varied aspects of nutrition and exercise, including sports. The topic of exercise and sports nutrition has been a focus of research among scientists since the 1960s, and the healthful benefits of good nutrition and exercise have been appreciated. As our knowledge expands, it will be necessary to remember that there must be a range of diets and exercise regimes that will support excellent physical condition and performance. There is not a single diet-exercise treatment that can be the common denominator, or the single formula for health, or panacea for performance.

This series is dedicated to providing a stage upon which to explore these issues. Each volume provides a detailed and scholarly examination of some aspect of the topic.

Contributors from any bona fide area of nutrition and physical activity, including sports and the controversial, are welcome.

I am pleased to welcome the contribution of *Nutrition and The Female Athlete* by my talented colleague Jaime S. Ruud.

Ira Wolinsky, Ph.D.

PREFACE

The purpose of this book is to provide current information related to nutrition and the female athlete. It is intended to reach a broad audience including female athletes, coaches, trainers, dietitians, and physicians.

Each chapter of this volume focuses on a topic of interest in the literature today. Chapter one begins with a brief overview of the nutrition knowlege and dietary practices of female athletes. It examines what female athletes know about nutrition, and some of the factors affecting their food choices. The results of dietary surveys of female athletes are summarized.

Chapter two covers the basic concepts of nutrition and how these concepts apply to sports nutrition. Dietary requirements for carbohydrates, protein, and fat are presented. Chapters three and four provide details on vitamins and minerals with special emphasis on the nutrients that are of particular importance to female athletes.

Chapter five presents the role of water and electrolytes, discussing the importance of consuming adequate fluids to prevent dehydration, and guidelines for optimal fluid replacement. Chapter six covers body weight and body composition, a topic of major concern to all female athletes. It examines factors affecting energy balance, and provides information on achieving a healthy competitive weight.

Finally, chapter seven provides an overview of eating disorders in athletes, including definition and diagnostic criteria, prevalence, risk factors, and effects on health and performance.

It is my hope that this book will offer scientific nutrition information in a way that is easy to understand, clear, and concise. This book was not meant to be comprehensive, but rather to serve as a "mini-course" on particular topics dealing with nutrition and the female athlete.

BIOGRAPHY

Jaime S. Ruud, M.S., R.D., is a nutrition consultant in private practice in Lincoln, NE. She graduated in 1975 from the University of Nebraska, with a degree in education and obtained her M.S. in Nutrition in 1979.

Since 1985 she has served as a consultant to the Center for Human Nutrition in Omaha, NE. She has co-authored and authored several chapters in books including, *Nutrition in Exercise and Sport, Nutrition for Women, Oxford Textbook of Medicine, Clinics in Sports Medicine, and Office Sports Medicine.* She has also written technical review papers for the U.S. Olympic Committee and articles for other publications.

She is a member of the American Dietetic Association, The American College of Sports Medicine, and The Society for Nutrition Education. She continues to devote her time to writing and consulting in nutrition and health.

ACKNOWLEDGMENTS

My sincerest thanks to my editor, Ira Wolinsky, who kept after me to write this book. I'm not sure this would have been possible without his encouragement, continued assistance, and great sense of humor.

I'd also like to gratefully acknowledge Ann Grandjean, Ed.D., who opened the window of opportunity for me in the field of sports nutrition. I wouldn't be where I am today without her guidance, expertise, and insight. Ann taught me three important principles of good writing: keep it short, keep it simple, and say it like it is.

A big thank you is also due to Sandy Wolfe Wood and Andrew Fuller for their graphic designs. The many individuals who provided technical support, including Colleen Holloran, Kathy Sundeen, Kathy Moore, Diane Kelley, and Anna Calhoun are also acknowledged.

Finally, I want to thank my family who put up with my strange hours, and my verbal expressions, "just a minute," and "I'm almost finished!"

Jaime S. Ruud, M.S., R.D.

TABLE OF CONTENTS

Chapter **1**

NUTRITION KNOWLEDGE AND PRACTICES OF FEMALE ATHLETES

CONTENTS

I. INTRODUCTION

As the number of women participating in athletics continues to grow, issues associated with the female athlete become increasingly important. Nutrition is one of the more important factors, but it is often misunderstood. Nutrition can impact performance in many ways. The well-nourished athlete has the energy and stamina to train hard and perform her best. Among comparable athletes, the one with the knowledge and practice of good nutrition most likely will have the competitive advantage.

Coaches, trainers, and health professionals should be aware of not only the nutritional requirements of women athletes, but also of the factors that influence dietary behaviors. Previous surveys[1-6] of nutrition knowledge and attitudes of female athletes have reported that:

1. There is a high level of interest in nutrition and a desire for more information.
2. Female athletes with prior nutrition education have higher nutrition knowledge and attitude scores but do not always apply this knowledge.
3. Weight control is a major factor influencing dietary practices of female athletes.

Indeed, female athletes may be more inclined to "eat right" if provided with appropriate information. However, gains in nutrition knowledge do not always translate into a behavior change.[7] For example, in a study of 31 female high school athletes, Perron and Endres[3] reported that 92% of the subjects knew milk was a good source of calcium but only 12% of the diets met the daily requirement for this mineral. Also, 81% of the female athletes reported that eating nutritious food was enjoyable, yet the largest portion of foods consumed over a 3-day period were carbonated drinks and concentrated sweets.

To be effective, nutrition education should focus on communicating information with a goal of influencing behavior.[8] The present system of nutrition education may be irrelevant to the needs of female athletes. Many of the guidelines used in the past, aimed at teaching the food groups, functions of nutrients in the body, and the science of nutrition are important objectives of nutrition education. However, we should determine what kind of nutrition information is reaching female athletes and how to improve upon this information so that it produces positive changes in eating habits. Presenting nutrition information from the perspective of how it relates to body weight and performance may be one way of reaching female athletes. More importantly, female athletes need a clearer understanding of how nutrition applies to them so that they can personalize their own eating plan, rather than simply follow general guidelines recommended for all athletes.

According to the "theory of meaningful learning," a principle that addresses education from a cognitive perspective, new knowledge is most effectively acquired when it is linked to concepts that the learner knows and believes are most important.[9] Updegrove and Achterberg[9] studied the meanings given to training and the role of eating in a group of high school distance runners. Results showed that "running" and "practice" were the most meaningful concepts related to training. "Coach" was the concept most often linked to eating. Thus, coaches are an important connection in the athlete's overall concept of nutrition, and they can influence an athlete's eating habits. Surveys[2,10] have reported that many coaches either lack a formal background in nutrition or are inadequately informed, indicating that this group should have access to more sports nutrition information.

II. FACTORS AFFECTING DIETARY PRACTICES OF FEMALE ATHLETES

Within a given population, there are different age groups, levels of education and income, and different audiences to be reached. Before nutrition messages can be communicated to female athletes, educators need to consider the factors affecting dietary intakes of female athletes, and they need to be aware of dietary problems and concerns.

Athletes eat for many different reasons: to increase energy, to build strength, to lose fat, to heal injuries, and to speed up recovery between training and competition. Many variables affect dietary practices of individuals, including physiological factors, food accessibility, environmental influences, and psychological factors.[11] Each of these factors determines the food choices athletes make (Figure 1.1).

Physiological Factors
Age, body size, sport, training intensity, menstrual cycle, pregnancy, lactation.

Food Accessibility
Availability, affordability.

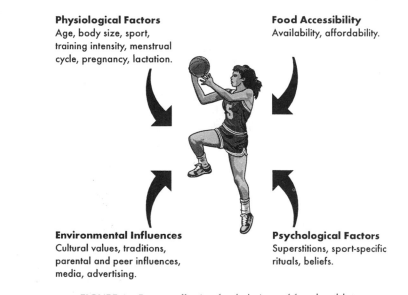

Environmental Influences
Cultural values, traditions, parental and peer influences, media, advertising.

Psychological Factors
Superstitions, sport-specific rituals, beliefs.

FIGURE 1 Factors affecting food choices of female athletes.

A. PHYSIOLOGICAL FACTORS

The physiological factors that affect an athlete's nutrient intake include age, sex, body size, type of sport, training routine, and duration and intensity of sport.[12] Additionally, hormonal changes during the menstrual cycle and pregnancy and lactation can alter the dietary patterns of women.

The physiological demands of specific sports vary widely and affect nutrient needs differently. For example, endurance athletes who train several hours a day need more calories to maintain energy levels, increased carbohydrate intake to maximize muscle glycogen stores, and adequate fluids to minimize dehydration.[13] Athletes participating in marathons, cycling, and triathlons are often unable to keep regular meal schedules and, therefore, rely on several small meals throughout the day.[14] For example, in a study by Lindeman,[15] triathletes ate an average of nine times a day. Snacks can contribute significantly to total daily intake. Butterworth et al.[16] studied food intake patterns of male and female marathon runners and found that snacks accounted for 29% of the caloric intake. As a result of continuously eating and drinking to meet energy demands, endurance athletes can experience more gastrointestinal problems such as heartburn, vomiting, bloating, and gas. These conditions can impair nutrient absorption and/or increase nutrient losses.[17]

In ballet, a dancer is required to achieve a desired body weight, usually 10 to 20% below her ideal weight.[18] To accomplish this goal, dancers often restrict calories and avoid foods like red meat and milk.[19] Additionally, their long practice hours significantly influence food choices. Cohen et al.[19] reported that during the dance season, members of the American Ballet Theater danced from 10:30 a.m. until 11 p.m. daily. No special time was set aside for lunch and half the dancers waited until after the last act to eat the major meal of the day. Diets were often monotonous and unbalanced. Sandri[20] reported that a dancer's daily diet may consist of one hard-boiled egg, plain lettuce, yogurt, vitamin supplements, and a diet beverage or coffee.

The physiological demands of bodybuilding greatly influence dietary practices and provide yet another example of how different sports affect eating behaviors and food choices. The bodybuilder strives to attain a low body fat level and a high degree of muscularity. Studies of female bodybuilders demonstrate dramatic changes in food intake, especially before competition.[21-23] Bodybuilders often exclude foods perceived to be high in fat, such as egg yolks, red meats, and most dairy products.[21] Their diets are often repetitive and lack variety.[22]

B. FOOD ACCESSIBILITY

Food accessibility refers to the availability and affordability of foods and is often determined by lifestyle and by living and working situations.[11] Most young athletes, who typically are fed by their parents or eat at school cafeterias, have little control over the type of foods that are purchased, prepared, and served to them.

Some college athletes live at home but most live on campus or in apartments. Many eat in university dining halls or at athletic training tables that serve at least one daily meal.[24] For athletes who do not live at home or on campus, cost becomes a major factor; many athletes simply cannot afford to spend a lot of money on food. They rely on convenience items or fast-foods because they are accessible, quick, and taste good.

C. ENVIRONMENTAL INFLUENCES

Cultural values, traditions, and parental and peer influences have a tremendous impact on eating habits. The desire to be thin influences the dietary practices of many young female athletes.[25] Unhealthy weight control methods can compromise strength and lead to decreased lean body mass, fatigue, and dehydration.[26]

Media and advertising greatly impact food choices of athletes. Visit almost any health food store and you'll find an ever-growing display of "sports nutrition" products, from protein powders and vitamin and mineral supplements to sports bars. Many female athletes turn to nutritional supplements as a means of losing weight or improving health and performance. Today, multivitamins are the most frequent type of nutritional supplement used by athletes, followed by vitamin C, iron, B-complex vitamins, and vitamin E.[27]

Television, along with magazine or newspaper articles about food and health, captures the interest of many athletes. According to Soper et al.,[28] professional magazines and newspapers and popular books, magazines, and nutrition labels were the most frequently reported sources of nutrition information among aerobic dance instructors. In another study,[29] 66% of the athletes' source of nutrition information came from television commercials, pamphlets, and nutrition labels. Athletes surveyed by Jacobson and Aldana[30] ranked popular magazines as the most prominent source of nutrition information. Popular magazines contain numerous advertisements for nutritional products, some of which are very misleading. According to Short and Marquart,[31] even the most informed athletes may not be able to predict the risks and/or benefits of the newest product hitting the market, nor perceive the long-term effects of using these products.

D. PSYCHOLOGICAL FACTORS

Educators should consider individual food preferences and the psychological implications behind them. Athletes may think that a specific food or meal will make them swim better, run faster, or jump higher. For example, one world-class cross country runner eats chocolate chip cookies before competition.[32] Many athletes have sport-specific rituals, superstitions, and/or routines involving foods that they believe will help them win. For instance, athletes in strength and power sports are concerned about protein sources and amino acid supplements. Endurance athletes, such as cyclists and runners often pursue dietary strategies that will increase carbohydrate stores in the body as well as effectively hydrate.[33] The psychological stresses of dieting to maintain low body weight greatly impact the eating habits of female athletes. Many weight-conscious athletes have developed a phobia about fat, both on their bodies and in their diets. Severely restricting fat and/or calories can lead to a myriad of nutrition-related health problems.[26] Female athletes need tailored nutrition messages on the healthy perspective of fat.

III. NUTRITION ASSESSMENT

After examining what female athletes know about nutrition and some of the factors affecting food choices, the next step is to gather dietary information. By doing so, educators can analyze what athletes are eating and identify nutritional problems.

Two methods frequently used to obtain dietary information are the 24-hour recall and the 3-day food intake record. The 24-hour recall relies on the individual's memory and motivation to recall the types and amounts of foods eaten in the past 24 hours. It is easy to administer and can provide estimates of individuals' usual intakes. One disadvantage is that a person's diet varies daily, so that a single day's intake may not represent actual dietary intake.[34] The 24-hour recall is also prone to over-reporting low intakes and under-reporting high intakes of some nutrients.[35-37]

The 3-day food intake record requires subjects to record everything they eat or drink for 3 or more days. Detailed instructions on how and when to record food intake are generally provided. Crawford et al.[38] found the 3-day food intake record more accurate than the 24-hour recall in assessing nutrient intake of young girls. In a nationwide survey of the nutritional habits of elite athletes, van Erp-Baart et al.[39] reported that, with a small number of subjects, recording for 4 days including the weekend provided more precise information than a 24-hour recall. However, de Vries et al.[40] found that 3-day food records underestimated energy intakes of young, well-educated adults.

Data obtained from nutrition surveys should allow researchers to draw conclusions about the dietary habits of athletes and the effect of nutrition on performance. But this is not feasible if the methods used to evaluate these factors are not valid and consistent. Future research should consider using larger sample sizes, collecting data at more frequent intervals over a longer period of time, and including sport-specific information.[41] Studies assessing the nutrient intake of female athletes should also include menstrual cycle variations and weight control practices.

The interpretation of dietary data assumes careful and complete record-keeping over a period of time.[42] It also depends on accurate food values and standards used to evaluate dietary data. *Bowes and Church's Food Values of Portions Commonly Used*[43] and the *U.S. Nutritive Value of Foods (U.S. Department of Agriculture Handbook No. 8)*[44] provide information on the nutrient content of foods. Most food composition data are collected from various sources (e.g., the food industry, scientific journals, trade journals, U.S. Department of Agriculture (USDA) publications); thus, limitations must be recognized.

Computer software programs also provide a variety of nutritional services, including nutrient analysis. Lee et al.[45] compared the general operating features and nutrient databases of eight microcomputer dietary analysis programs. The programs varied in cost, number of foods and nutrients in the database, use of non-USDA data, and substitution of data for missing values. According to Lee et al.,[45] when choosing a dietary analysis program, one of the most important considerations is the database. It must be accurate, well documented, and large enough to perform the specific tasks.[45]

A. RECOMMENDED DIETARY ALLOWANCES

The Recommended Dietary Allowances (RDA) are the standards most commonly used in the U.S. for evaluating the nutrient intakes of populations and for planning diets.[46] Established by the Food and Nutrition Board of the National Academy of Sciences, the RDAs are defined as "the levels of intake of essential nutrients that, on the basis of scientific knowledge, are judged by the Food and Nutrition board to be adequate to meet the known nutrient needs of practically all healthy persons."[46] They are neither minimal amounts nor optimal amounts, but rather are safe and adequate levels that include a generous margin of safety. The safety factor established for each nutrient reflects current knowledge of individual differences, bioavailability (the total amount of nutrient available for absorption), and changes in the food supply.[46]

The RDAs include recommendations for protein, 11 vitamins, and seven minerals (Table 1.1). No RDA is set for carbohydrate or fat. Additionally, estimated safe and adequate intakes are provided in ranges for selected vitamins, minerals, and energy (Table 1.2). Because nutritional requirements vary with age, sex, body size, and physiological state, the RDAs are presented for males and females in different age and weight groups.

Although the RDAs are recommended average daily intakes set high enough to ensure that nutrient needs are met, they do not necessarily cover each individual for every nutrient. When analyzing dietary data, one should not equate nutrient intakes below 100% of the RDA with nutritional deficiency. However, nutrient intakes less than two-thirds (67%) of the RDA are often used as a cut-off point for "less than adequate" intakes in dietary surveys, including research involving athletes.[4,47-49]

The RDAs are reviewed periodically and recommendations are made based on new research and new interpretations. In the 10th edition of the RDAs, published in 1989, some major changes were made (Table 1.3):

- The RDA for vitamin K and selenium are established for the first time.
- The allowances for vitamin B_6, folate, and vitamin B_{12} are lower than in previous editions based upon current research.
- Calcium is set at 1200 mg/d for ages 11 to 24. The subcommittee has extended this allowance through age 24 because of studies demonstrating that attainment of peak bone mass occurs after age 18.
- The allowances for the minerals iron and zinc are reduced for women.

There is considerable debate on whether the RDAs are appropriate for use with athletes. First, the RDAs are expressed in terms of "reference individuals," so adjustments must be made for athletes with a body mass significantly different from the average male or female. Second, the RDAs do not

TABLE 1.1 Recommended Dietary Allowances (For Females)

Age (Years)	Children 7–10	Females 11–14	15–18	19–24	25–50	51+	Pregnant	Lactating First Trimester	Second Trimester
Weight									
(kg)	28	46	55	58	63	65			
(lb)	62	101	120	128	138	143			
Height									
(cm)	132	157	163	164	163	160			
(in)	52	62	64	65	64	63			
Protein									
(g)	28	46	44	46	50	50	60	65	62
Fat soluble vitamins									
Vitamin A (µg RE)	700	800	800	800	800	800	800	1300	1200
Vitamin D (µg)	10	10	10	10	5	5	10	10	10
Vitamin K (µg)	30	45	55	60	65	65	65	65	65
Vitamin E (mg α-TE)	7	8	8	8	8	8	10	12	11

Water soluble vitamins									
Vitamin C (mg)	45	50	60	60	60	60	70	95	90
Thiamin (mg)	1.0	1.1	1.1	1.1	1.1	1.0	1.5	1.6	1.6
Riboflavin (mg)	1.2	1.3	1.3	1.3	1.3	1.2	1.6	1.8	1.7
Niacin (mg NE)	13	15	15	15	15	13	17	20	20
Vitamin B_6 (mg)	1.4	1.4	1.5	1.6	1.6	1.6	2.2	2.1	2.1
Folate (µg)	100	150	180	180	180	180	400	280	260
Vitamin B_{12} (µg)	1.4	2.0	2.0	2.0	2.0	2.0	2.2	2.6	2.6
Minerals									
Calcium (mg)	800	1200	1200	1200	800	800	1200	1200	1200
Phosphorus (mg)	800	1200	1200	1200	800	800	1200	1200	1200
Magnesium (mg)	170	280	300	280	280	280	320	355	340
Iron (mg)	10	15	15	15	15	10	30	15	15
Zinc (mg)	10	12	12	12	12	12	15	19	16
Iodine (µg)	120	150	150	150	150	150	175	200	200
Selenium (µg)	30	45	50	55	55	55	65	75	75

Adapted from the Food and Nutrition Board, National Research Council, *Recommended Dietary Allowances*, 10th ed., National Academy Press, Washington, D.C., 1989.

TABLE 1.2   Estimated Safe and Adequate Daily Dietary Intakes of Selected Vitamins and Minerals

Age (Years)	Children and Adolescents		Adults
	7–10	11+	
Vitamins			
Biotin (µg)	30	30–100	30–100
Pantothenic acid (mg)	4–5	4–7	4–7
Trace elements			
Copper (mg)	1.0–2.0	1.5–2.5	1.5–3.0
Manganese (mg)	2.0–3.0	2.0–5.0	2.0–5.0
Fluoride (mg)	1.5–2.5	1.5–2.5	1.5–4.0
Chromium (µg)	50–200	50–200	50–200
Molybdenum (µg)	50–150	75–250	75–250

Adapted from the Food and Nutrition Board, National Research Council, *Recommended Dietary Allowances,* 10th ed., National Academy Press, Washington, D.C., 1989.

TABLE 1.3   Changes in the Tenth Edition of the RDAs (For Females)

Nutrient	1980	1989
Selenium (µg)	No RDA	55
Vitamin K (µg/kg BW)	No RDA	1
Vitamin B_6 (mg)	2.0	1.6
Folate (µg)	400	180
Vitamin B_{12} (µg)	3	2
Iron (mg)	18	15
Zinc (mg)	15	12
Calcium (mg)	1200	1200
	through age 18	through age 24
Protein (g)		
During pregnancy	30	60
Vitamin C (mg)		
During pregnancy	60	70
Magnesium (mg)		
During pregnancy	150	320
During lactation	150	355

Adapted from the Food and Nutrition Board, National Research Council, *Recommended Dietary Allowances,* 10th ed., National Academy Press, Washington, D.C., 1989.

take into consideration the demands of strenuous activity. Protein is one example. Research shows that prolonged exercise increases the oxidation of protein, and under certain conditions, such as decreased muscle glycogen, total oxidation can become significant.[50] Nitrogen balance studies indicate that endurance and strength-trained athletes need more than the RDA of 0.8 g protein/kg bw/d. Sport scientists now recommend a protein intake between 1.2 and 1.8 g protein/kg bw/d.[51] Finally, the RDAs do not apply to individuals who exercise in hot environments. Prolonged exercise in the heat increases water and sodium losses through sweat and may lead to measurable losses of essential nutrients such as potassium, iron, and zinc. Thus, these factors should be considered when applying the RDAs to athletes.

Despite limitations and until more data become available, the RDAs are the only standards for evaluating the nutrient intake of populations, including athletes.

IV. DIETARY SURVEYS OF FEMALE ATHLETES

It has been said that dietary surveys of athletes are useful not to set standards of nutrition but rather to discover deficiencies and thus know what dietary corrections are needed.[52] When reviewing dietary data, comparisons of athletes' nutrient intakes should consider, when possible, differences in methodology, sample size, level of competition (amateur, collegiate, elite), and manner in which dietary information is reported.

The results of dietary surveys of female athletes from a variety of sports were reviewed and are summarized in Table 1.4. The majority of these studies were conducted between 1985 and 1995 and used 3-day food records to collect dietary data. Studies conducted prior to 1989 analyzed and compared data with the 1980 RDAs, so mean nutrients intakes should be examined carefully.

A. ENERGY INTAKES

As can be seen in Table 1.4, there is a wide range of energy intakes for female athletes both within and between sport groups. Female triathletes, swimmers, and heavyweight rowers had among the highest mean daily energy intakes ranging from 2633 kcal/d to 4149 kcal/d. The lowest mean energy intakes were noted for female bodybuilders during competition (1249 kcal/d), gymnasts (1381 to 2298 kcal/d), and dancers (1673 to 1890 kcal/d). Although not provided here because of lack of data, reporting energy intake on a body weight basis is more representative of actual energy intakes. For example, the absolute mean energy intake of female gymnasts studied by Reggiani et al.[65] was significantly lower than the recommended dietary allowance of 2200 kcal/d for females ages 11 to 18.[46] However, when calculated on a body weight basis, the gymnasts averaged 43 kcal/kg which is within a normal range (40 to 47 kcal/kg).

Based on the studies reported here, mean energy intakes of female athletes are often marginal. Female athletes participating in endurance sports, such as running, cycling, and swimming would be expected to increase energy intake to meet the additional demands of training and competition. According to Economos et al.,[53] a female athlete weighing 55 kg (121 lb) and expending

TABLE 1.4 Mean Nutrient Intakes of Female Athletes

Sport Group	No.	Age	Energy (kcal)	Protein (g)	Protein %	Cho (g)	Cho %	Fat (g)	Fat %	Iron mg	Calc mg	Zinc mg	Vit B6 mg	Folate µg
Runners														
Bergen-Cico and Short[54]	44	13	2,488	—	15	—	49	—	34	12.4	972	9.0	1.0	168
Deuster et al.[a55]	51	29	2,397	80	—	322	—	89	—	41.9	1,227	14.2	—	—
Kaiserauer et al.[56]	9	26	2,490	86	—	180	48	95	38	12.9	1,200	10.2	2.1	276
Manore et al.[57]	10	34	2,272	77	14	272	—	95	—	13.7	—	—	1.8	252
Nieman et al.[58]	56	37	1,868	73	—	246	48	86	31	14.2	797	8.2	1.6	266
Pate et al.[59]	103	30	1,603	—	15	192	—	57	—	11.2	630	6.7	1.3	—
Schemmel et al.[60]	15	15	2,258	78	—	—	—	88	—	—	—	—	—	—
Tanaka et al.[61]	10	19	1,988	64	13	331	67	50	22	—	—	—	—	—
Cyclists														
Keith et al.[48]	8	22	1,781	64	14	264	60	57	26	10.6	719	7.2	—	303
Gymnasts														
Benardot et al.[62]	22	13	1,706	67	15	227	52	62	32	11.0	867	—	—	—
Benson et al.[63]	12	12	1,544	65	17	—	53	—	30	10.4	966	—	1.5	242
Chen et al.[64]	5	18	2,298	94	16	242	42	106	42	36.0	807	—	—	—
Kirchner et al.[47]	26	19	1,381	53	—	180	—	47	—	11.8	683	—	—	—
Loosli et al.[4]	97	13	1,838	71	15	220	49	74	36	—	—	—	—	—
Moffatt[66]	13	15	1,923	74	15	221	46	81	38	11.2	706	7.4	1.3	129
Reggiani et al.[65]	26	12	1,552	61	15	—	47	—	36	6.2	539	—	0.6	38
Triathletes														
Green et al.[14]	34	—	4,149	113	11	695	66	99	21	—	—	—	—	—
Khoo et al.[67]	10	38	2,474	80	—	351	—	85	—	—	—	—	—	—

Swimmers													
Barr[69]	10	16	2,064	89	—	284	—	69	—	15.6	1,354	9.3	1.8	—
Barr[68]	14	19	2,296	73	—	324	—	82	—	14.7	808	—	—	—
Benson et al.[63]	18	12	1,892	66	14	—	51	—	35	10.1	764	—	1.2	159
Berning et al.[70]	21	15	3,572	107	12	428	47	164	41	18.3	1,234	—	—	—
Tilgner and Schiller[71]	19	19	2,493	79	—	337	—	91	—	13.2	1,046	6.7	—	248
Vallieres et al.[72]	6	22	2,472	90	—	333	—	93	—	13.3	970	—	—	—
Dancers													
Benson et al.[76]	92	14	1,890	72	15	235	49	75	34	13.4	932	7.6	1.6	266
Cohen et al.[19]	12	24	1,673	59	14	206	50	71	38	13.5	821	—	0.9	67
Evers[77]	21	21	1,775	59	—	—	—	—	—	10.0	953	—	—	—
Basketball													
Nowak et al.[73]	10	19	1,730	68	—	229	—	63	—	10.0	903	7.0	1.0	173
Hockey Players													
Tilgner and Schiller[71]	8	19	1,956	76	—	228	—	87	—	10.5	762	6.8	—	127
Heavyweight Rowers													
Steen et al.[74]	16	21	2,633	88	13	337	51	104	36	—	—	—	—	—
Field Athletes													
Faber and Spinnler Benade[49]	10	22	2,215	—	17	—	46	—	38	13.3	739	13.1	1.6	230
Bodybuilders[b]													
Heyward et al.[75]	25	28	1,453	77	21	261	72	15	10	11.3	271	7.4	—	—
Kleiners et al.[23]	8	28	2,260	162	37	332	49	33	13	24	293	9.0	—	—
Lamar-Hildebrand et al.[21]	10	18–30	1,249	76	—	196	—	21	—	14	390	—	—	—

a   Includes food and supplements
b   Preparing for competition

approximately 800 to 1200 kcal/d during training would require between 2600 and 3300 kcal/d. Low energy intakes may reflect weight control practices of female athletes.

B. ENERGY DISTRIBUTION

The studies summarized in Table 1.4 revealed great variance in the distribution of energy from protein, carbohydrates, and fat. Overall mean intakes of protein ranged from 12 to 37%, carbohydrates from 42 to 72%, and fat from 10 to 42%. The runners, cyclists, and triathletes generally consumed a greater percentage of energy from carbohydrates (48 to 67%) than other sport groups. More recently, scientists have begun reporting carbohydrate and protein as grams per kilogram body weight which allows for a more accurate description.

Mean fat intakes ranged from 10% for championship female bodybuilders during competition to 42% for amateur female gymnasts. Female runners studied by Tanaka et al.,[61] triathletes studied by Green et al.,[14] and cyclists studied by Keith et al.[48] had low mean fat intakes (21 to 25% of kcal). However, most sport groups consumed between 34 and 38% of calories from fat.

C. VITAMINS AND MINERALS

Because few studies provide analysis of all vitamins and minerals, those that have frequently been reported to be low in diets of female athletes were included in this review. They include iron, calcium, zinc, vitamin B_6, and folate.

With the exception of female swimmers studied by Berning et al.,[70] and runners studied by Deuster et al.,[55] the majority of sport groups had mean iron intakes below the 15 mg/d recommended for females ages 11 to 51.[46] Mean dietary intakes of calcium, zinc, and vitamin B_6 were also frequently lower than the RDAs of 1200 mg/d, 12 mg/d, and 1.6 mg/d, respectively. The studies reviewed here further support the concept that female athletes with low energy intakes also tend to have low intakes of essential vitamins and minerals (Table 1.5).

V. CONCLUSIONS

Although many factors affect the dietary practices of female athletes, the desire to be thin has the greatest impact. Educators need to determine what type of information is reaching female athletes and improve upon this information so it produces positive changes in eating habits. Presenting nutrition information from the perspective of how it relates to body weight and performance may be an effective way to reach female athletes.

Dietary surveys suggest that the diets of many female athletes are lower in carbohydrate and higher in fat than recommended for health and performance.[52] Studies also reveal that female athletes are not consuming enough

TABLE 1.5   Nutritional Problems of Female Athletes

Sport Group

Runners
Bergen-Cico and Short[54]	Low dietary intakes of B_6, calcium, zinc, low carbohydrate intake
Deuster et al.[55]	Low dietary intakes of zinc, iron
Kaiserauer et al.[56]	Low carbohydrate intake, low dietary intakes of iron, zinc
Manore et al.[57]	Low dietary intake of iron, low carbohydrate intake
Nieman et al.[58]	Low energy intake, low dietary intakes of iron, calcium, zinc, vitamin B_6
Pate et al.[59]	Low energy intake, low carbohydrate intake, low dietary intakes of iron, calcium, zinc, vitamin B_6
Schemmel et al.[60]	Low dietary intake of iron
Tanaka et al.[61]	Low energy intake

Cyclists
Keith et al.[48]	Low energy intake, low dietary intakes of calcium, zinc

Gymnasts
Benardot et al.[62]	Low dietary intakes of iron, calcium
Benson et al.[63]	Low energy intake, low dietary intakes of vitamin B_6, calcium, iron
Chen et al.[64]	Low carbohydrate intake, higher fat intake, low dietary intake of calcium
Kirchner et al.[47]	Low energy intake, low carbohydrate intake, low dietary intakes of calcium, iron
Loosli et al.[4]	Low energy intake
Moffatt[66]	Low energy intake, low dietary intakes of calcium, folate, vitamin B_6, iron, zinc
Reggiani et al.[65]	Low energy intake, low dietary intakes of vitamin B_6, calcium, iron, folate

Swimmers
Barr[69]	Low dietary intake of zinc
Barr[68]	Low dietary intake of calcium
Benson et al.[63]	Low energy intake, low dietary intakes of iron, calcium, vitamin B_6, folate
Berning et al.[70]	Higher fat intake, low carbohydrate intake
Tilgner and Schiller[71]	Low dietary intakes of iron, zinc
Vallieres et al.[72]	Low dietary intakes of iron, calcium

Dancers
Benson et al.[76]	Low energy intake, low dietary intakes of iron, calcium, zinc, and vitamin B_6
Cohen et al.[19]	Low energy intake, low dietary intakes of vitamin B_6, iron, calcium, folate
Evers[77]	Low energy intake, low dietary intake of iron, calcium

Basketball
Nowak et al.[73]	Low energy intake, low dietary intakes of iron, calcium, zinc, vitamin B_6, folate

Hockey players
Tilgner and Schiller[71]	Low energy intake, low dietary intakes of iron, calcium, zinc

Heavyweight rowers
Steen et al.[74]	Low carbohydrate intake, low dietary intakes of vitamin B_6, calcium, zinc

TABLE 1.5 (continued)   Nutritional Problems of Female Athletes

Sport Group

Field athletes
  Faber and Spinnler Benade[49]   Low dietary intake of iron, calcium, vitamin B$_6$, higher fat
                                   intake
Bodybuilders
  Heyward et al.[75]   Low energy intake, low dietary fat intake, low dietary intakes
                                   of iron, calcium, zinc
  Kleiner et al.[23]   Low dietary fat intake, high protein intake, low dietary intakes
                                   of calcium, zinc
  Lamar-Hildebrand et al.[21]   Low energy intake, low dietary fat intake, low calcium intake

energy to support their activity level. As energy intake decreases, so does nutrient intake, which is reflected in their low intakes of vitamins and minerals, particularly iron, calcium, zinc, vitamin B$_6$, and folate. Low energy and nutrient intakes place female athletes at greater risk for nutrition-related problems such as amenorrhea, decreased bone density, iron deficiency anemia, and eating disorders, all of which can have an adverse effect on health and performance. Information on these topics is presented throughout this book.

REFERENCES

1. Werblow, J. A., Fox, H. M., and Henneman, A., Nutritional knowledge, attitudes, and food patterns of women athletes, *J. Am. Diet. Assoc.*, 73, 242, 1978.
2. Parr, R. B., Porter, M. A., and Hodgson, S. C., Nutrition knowledge and practice of coaches, trainers, and athletes, *Phys. Sportmed.*, 12, 127, 1984.
3. Perron, M. and Endres, J., Knowledge, attitudes, and dietary practices of female athletes, *J. Am. Diet. Assoc.*, 85, 573, 1985.
4. Loosli, A. R., Benson, J., Gillien, D. M., and Bourdet, K., Nutrition habits and knowledge in competitive adolescent female gymnasts, *Phys. Sportsmed.*, 14, 118, 1986.
5. Welch, P. K., Zager, K. A., Endres, J., and Poon, S. W., Nutrition education, body composition, and dietary intake of female college athletes, *Phys. Sportsmed.*, 15, 63, 1987.
6. Short, S. H., Surveys of dietary intake and nutrition knowledge of athletes and their coaches, in *Nutrition in Exercise and Sport*, Wolinsky, I. and Hickson, J. F., Eds., CRC Press, Inc., Boca Raton, 1994, 367.
7. Potter, G. S. and Wood, O. B., Comparison of self and group instruction for teaching sports nutrition to college athletes, *J. Nutr. Educ.*, 23, 288, 1991.
8. Guthrie, H. A., Is education not enough? *J. Nutr. Educ.*, 910, 57, 1978.
9. Updegrove, N. A. and Achterberg, C. L., The conceptual relationship between training and eating in high school distance runners, *J. Nutr. Educ.*, 23, 18, 1990.
10. Graves, K. L., Farthing, M. C., Smith, S. A., and Turchi, J. M., Nutrition training, attitudes, knowledge, recommendations, responsibility, and resource utilization of high school coaches and trainers, *J. Am. Diet. Assoc.*, 91, 321, 1991.
11. Pennington, J. A. T., Dietary patterns and practices, *Clin. Nutr.*, 5, 17, 1986.
12. Storlie, J., Nutrition assessment of athletes: A model for integrating nutrition and physical performance indicators, *Int. J. Sport Nutr.*, 1, 192, 1991.
13. Costill, D. L. and Miller, J. M., Nutrition for endurance sport: carbohydrate and fluid balance, *Int. J. Sports Med.*, 1, 2, 1980.

14. Green, D. R., Gibbons, C., O'Toole, M., Hiller, W. B. O., An evaluation of dietary intakes of triathletes: Are RDAs being met?, *J. Am. Diet. Assoc.,* 89, 1653, 1989.
15. Lindeman, A. K., Eating and training habits of triathletes: A balancing act, *J. Am. Diet. Assoc.,* 90, 993, 1990.
16. Butterworth, D. E., Nieman, D. C., Butler, J. V., and Herring, J. L., Food intake patterns of marathon runners, *Int. J. Sport Nutr.,* 4, 1, 1994.
17. Worme, J. D., Doubt, T. J., Singh, A., Ryan, C. J., Moses, F. M., and Deuster, P. A., Dietary patterns, gastrointestinal complaints, and nutrition knowledge of recreational triathletes, *Am. J. Clin. Nutr.,* 51, 690, 1990.
18. Hamilton, W. G., Warren, M. P., and Hamilton, L. H., Physical and psychological aspects of dance medicine, *Kinesiol. Med. Dance,* 16, 12, 1993–94.
19. Cohen, J. L., Potosnak, L., Frank, O., and Baker, H., A nutritional and hematologic assessment of elite ballet dancers, *Phys. Sportsmed.,* 13, 43, 1985.
20. Sandri, S. C., On dancers and diet, *Int. J. Sport Nutr.,* 3, 334, 1993.
21. Lamar-Hildebrand, N., Saldanha, L., and Endres, J., Dietary and exercise practices of college-aged female bodybuilders, *J. Am. Diet. Assoc.,* 89, 1308, 1989.
22. Sandoval, W. M. and Heyward, V. H., Food selection patterns of bodybuilders, *Int. J. Sport Nutr.,* 1, 61, 1991.
23. Kleiner, S. M., Bazzarre, T. L., and Litchford, M. D., Metabolic profiles, diet, and health practices of championship male and female bodybuilders, *J. Am. Diet. Assoc.,* 90, 962, 1990.
24. Clark, K. L., Working with college athletes, coaches, and trainers at a major university, *Int. J. Sport Nutr.,* 4, 135, 1994.
25. Nutter, J., Seasonal changes in female athletes' diets, *Int. J. Sport Nutr.,* 1, 395, 1991.
26. Pugliese, M. T., Lifshitz, F., Grad, G., Fort, P., and Marks-Katz, M., Fear of obesity: a cause of short stature and delayed puberty, *N. Engl. J. Med.,* 309, 513, 1983.
27. Sobal, J. and Marquart, L. F., Vitamin/mineral supplement use among athletes: A review of the literature, *Int. J. Sport Nutr.,* 4, 320, 1994.
28. Soper, J., Carpenter, R. A., and Shannon, B. M., Nutrition knowledge of aerobic dance instructors, *J. Nutr. Educ.,* 24, 59, 1992.
29. Barr, S. I., Nutrition knowledge and selected nutritional practices of female recreational athletes, *J. Nutr. Educ.,* 18, 167, 1986.
30. Jacobson, B. H. and Aldana, S. G., Current nutrition practice and knowledge of varsity athletes, *J. Appl. Sport Sci. Res.,* 6, 232, 1992.
31. Short, S. H. and Marquart, L. F., Sports nutrition fraud, *N.Y. State J. Med.,* 93, 112, 1993.
32. Kuehls, D., Very superstitious, *Runners World,* 39, Oct., 1994.
33. Singh, A., Pelletier, P. A., and Deuster, P. A., Dietary requirements for ultra-endurance exercise, *Sports Med.,* 18, 301, 1994.
34. Dwyer, J. T., Dietary assessment, in *Modern Nutrition In Health and Disease,* 8th ed., Shils, M. E., Olson, J. A., and Shike, M., Eds., Lea & Febiger, Philadelphia, 1994, 842.
35. Karvetti, R. L. and Knuts, L. R., Validity of the 24-hour dietary recall, *J. Am. Diet. Assoc.,* 85, 1437, 1985.
36. Gersovitz, M., Madden, J. P., and Smiciklas-Wright, H., Validity of the 24-hour dietary recall and seven-day record for group comparisons, *J. Am. Diet. Assoc.,* 73, 48, 1978.
37. Carter, R. L., Sharbaugh, C. O., and Stapell, C. A., Reliability and validity of the 24-hour recall, *J. Am. Diet. Assoc.,* 79, 542, 1981.
38. Crawford, P. B., Obarzanek, E., Morrison, J., and Sabry, Z. I., Comparative advantage of 3-day food records over 24-hour recall and 5-day food frequency validated by observation of 9- and 10-year-old girls, *J. Am. Diet. Assoc.,* 94, 626, 1994.
39. van Erp-Baart, A. M. J., Saris, W. H. M., Binkhorst, R. A., Vos, J. A., and Elvers, J. W. H., Nationwide survey on nutritional habits in elite athletes. Part I. Energy, carbohydrate, protein, and fat intake, *Int. J. Sports Med.,* 10, Suppl 1, S3, 1989.

40. de Vries, J. H. M., Zock, P. L., Mensink, R. P., and Katan, M. B., Underestimation of energy intake by 3-d records compared with energy intake to maintain body weight in 269 nonobese adults, *Am. J. Clin. Nutr.*, 60, 855, 1994.

41. Grandjean, A. C. and Ruud, J. S., Energy intake of athletes, in *Oxford Textbook of Sports Medicine*, Harris, M., Williams, C., Stanish, W. D., and Micheli, L. J., Eds., Oxford University Press, New York, 1994, 53.

42. Guthrie, H. A., Interpretation of data on dietary intake. *Nutr. Rev.*, 47, 33, 1989.

43. Pennington, J. A. T., *Bowes & Church's Food Values of Portions Commonly Used*, 16th ed., J. B. Lippincott Company, Philadelphia, 1994.

44. United States Department of Agriculture, Human Nutrition Information Service, *Nutritive Value of Foods,* Home and Garden Bulletin No. 72, 1991.

45. Lee, R. D., Nieman, D. C., and Rainwater, M., Comparison of eight microcomputer dietary analysis programs with the USDA nutrient data base for standard reference, *J. Am. Diet. Assoc.*, 95, 858, 1995.

46. Food and Nutrition Board, National Research Council, *Recommended Dietary Allowances*, 10th ed., National Academy Press, Washington, D.C., 1989.

47. Kirchner, E. M., Lewis, R. D., and O'Connor, P. J., Bone mineral density and dietary intake of female college gymnasts, *Med. Sci. Sports Exerc.*, 27, 543, 1995.

48. Keith, R. E., O'Keeffe, K. A., Alt, L. A., and Young, K. L., Dietary status of trained female cyclists, *J. Am. Diet. Assoc.*, 89, 1620, 1989.

49. Faber, M. and Spinnler Benade, A. J., Mineral and vitamin intake in field athletes (discus, hammer, javelin-throwers and shotputters), *Int. J. Sports Med.*, 12, 324, 1991.

50. Lemon, P. W. R. and Nagle, F. J., Effects of exercise on protein and amino acid metabolism, *Med. Sci. Sports Exerc.*, 13, 141, 1981.

51. Lemon, P. W. R. Do athletes need more dietary protein and amino acids? *Int. J. Sport Nutr.*, 5, S39, 1995.

52. Leaf, A. and Frisa, K. B., Eating for health or for athletic performance? *Am. J. Clin. Nutr.*, 49, 1066, 1989.

53. Economos, C. D., Bortz, S. S., and Nelson, M. E., Nutritional practices of elite athletes, *Sports Med.*, 16, 381, 1993.

54. Bergen-Cico, D. K. and Short, S. H., Dietary intakes, energy expenditures, and anthropometric characteristics of adolescent female cross-country runners, *J. Am. Diet. Assoc.*, 92, 611, 1992.

55. Deuster, P. A., Kyle, S. B., Moser, P. B., Vigersky, R. A., Singh, A., and Schoomaker, E. B., Nutritional survey of highly trained women runners, *Am. J. Clin. Nutr.*, 44, 954, 1986.

56. Kaiserauer, S., Snyder, A. C., Sleeper, M., and Zierath, J., Nutritional, physiological, and menstrual status of distance runners, *Med. Sci. Sports Exerc.*, 21, 120, 1989.

57. Manore, M. M., Besenfelder, P. D., Wells, C. L., Carroll, S. S., and Hooker, S. P., Nutrient intakes and iron status in female long-distance runners during training, *J. Am. Diet. Assoc.*, 89, 257, 1989.

58. Nieman, D. C., Bulter, J. V., Pollett, L. M., Dietrich, S. J., and Lutz, R. D., Nutrient intake of marathon runners, *J. Am. Diet. Assoc.*, 89, 1273, 1989.

59. Pate, R. R., Sargent, R. G., Baldwin, C., and Burgess, M. L., Dietary intake of women runners, *Int. J. Sports Med.*, 11, 461, 1990.

60. Schemmel, R. A., Stone, M., and Conn, C., Comparison of dietary habits and nutrient intake of competitive runners with age- and gender-matched controls, in *Sport For Children and Youths*, Weiss, M. R., and Gould, D., Eds., Human Kinetics, Champaign, 1986, 231.

61. Tanaka, J. A., Tanaka, H., and Landis, W., An assessment of carbohydrate intake in collegiate distance runners, *Int. J. Sport Nutr.*, 5, 206, 1995.

62. Benardot, D., Schwarz, M., and Heller, D. W., Nutrient intake in young, highly competitive gymnasts, *J. Am. Diet. Assoc.*, 89, 401, 1989.

63. Benson, J. E., Allemann, Y., Theintz, G. E., and Howald, H., Eating problems and calorie intake levels in Swiss adolescent athletes, *Int. J. Sports Med.*, 11, 249, 1990.

64. Chen, J. D., Wang, J. F., Li, K. J., Zhao, Y. W., Jiao, Y., and Hou, X. Y., Nutritional problems and measures in elite and amateur athletes, *Am. J. Clin. Nutr.*, 49, 1084, 1989.

65. Reggiani, E., Arras, G. B., Trabacca, S., Senarega, D., and Chiodini, G., Nutritional status and body composition of adolescent female gymnasts, *J. Sports Med.*, 29, 285, 1989.

66. Moffatt, R. J., Dietary status of elite female high school gymnasts: inadequacy of vitamin and mineral intake, *J. Am. Diet. Assoc.*, 84, 1361, 1984.

67. Khoo, Chor-San, Rawson, N. E., Robinson, M. L., and Stevenson, R. J., Nutrient intake and eating habits of triathletes, *Ann. Sports Med.*, 3, 144, 1987.

68. Barr, S. I., Relationship of eating attitudes to anthropometric variables and dietary intakes of female collegiate swimmers, *J. Am. Diet. Assoc.*, 91, 976, 1991.

69. Barr, S. I., Energy and nutrient intakes of elite adolescent swimmers, *J. Can. Diet. Assoc.*, 50, 20, 1989.

70. Berning, J. R., Troup, J. P., VanHandel, P. J., Daniels, J., and Daniels, N., The nutritional habits of young adolescent swimmers, *Int. J. Sport Nutr.*, 1, 240, 1991.

71. Tilgner, S. A. and Schiller, M. R., Dietary intakes of female college athletes: the need for nutrition education, *J. Am. Diet. Assoc.*, 89, 967, 1989.

72. Vallieres, F., Tremblay, A., and St-Jean, L., Study of the energy balance and the nutritional status of highly trained female swimmers, *Nutr. Res.*, 9, 699, 1989.

73. Nowak, R. K., Knudsen, K. S., and Schultz, L. O., Body composition and nutrient intakes of college men and women basketball players, *J. Am. Diet. Assoc.*, 88, 575, 1988.

74. Steen, S. N., Mayer, K., Brownell, K. D., and Wadden, T. A., Dietary intake of female collegiate heavyweight rowers, *Int. J. Sport Nutr.*, 5, 225, 1995.

75. Heyward, V. H., Sandoval, W. M., and Colville, B. C., Anthropometric, body composition and nutritional profiles of bodybuilders during training, *J. Appl. Sport Sci. Res.*, 3, 22, 1989.

76. Benson, J. E., Gillien, D. M., Bourdet, K., and Loosli, A. R., Inadequate nutrition and chronic calorie restriction in adolescent ballerinas, *Phys. Sportsmed.*, 13, 79, 1985.

77. Evers, C. L., Dietary intake and symptoms of anorexia nervosa in female university dancers, *J. Am. Diet. Assoc.*, 87, 66, 1987.

Chapter 2

THE ENERGY YIELDING NUTRIENTS: CARBOHYDRATES, PROTEIN, AND FAT

CONTENTS

I. INTRODUCTION

Nutrition is the study of food in relation to health. Most simply, it is the food we eat and how our body uses it. A more comprehensive definition of nutrition has been developed by the Food and Nutrition Council of the American Medical Association.[1] "Nutrition is the science of food, the nutrients and other substances therein, their action, interaction and balance in relation to health and disease, and the processes by which the organism ingests, digests, absorbs, transports, utilizes and excretes food substances."

The study of nutrition is about 200 years old. However, sports nutrition is a relatively new discipline involving the application of nutritional principles to enhance athletic performance.[2] It has evolved at least in part from its parent discipline, sports medicine. As an independent discipline, sports nutrition is still in the formative stage. It is practiced in a variety of settings by people from a variety of disciplines who subspecialize in this field.[3]

Nutrition affects an athlete in many ways. At the basic level, it plays an important role in achieving and maintaining health. Optimal nutrition can reduce fatigue, allowing an athlete to train and compete longer or recover faster between training sessions. It can also reduce susceptibility to disease and injury. However, good nutrition by itself cannot guarantee well-being and athletic success. Other factors that influence health and performance include the amount of sleep an athlete gets, genetic predisposition to certain diseases, protection from excessive environmental and psychological stresses, and good medical care.[4]

II. BASICS OF NUTRITION

The basic concepts of nutrition were developed over 30 years ago and have been used by nutrition educators to help individuals make decisions about food. Today, these same concepts can be applied to sports nutrition. They are as follows:

1. Nutrition is the food you eat and how your body uses it.
   Athletes need food to live, to grow, and to stay healthy. The well-nourished athlete has more energy and strength than the undernourished athlete and thus is able to train harder and recover faster from exercise.

2. Food is made up of different nutrients for growth and health.

   Every nutrient required by the body can be supplied through food. The body needs more than 40 nutrients every day. These nutrients come from protein, carbohydrates, fats, vitamins, minerals, and water. No single food or supplement can provide all the nutrients necessary for growth and health. A variety of foods are needed every day, but many different dietary patterns can provide good nutrition. Each nutrient has specific uses in the body. Most nutrients function optimally in the body when teamed with other nutrients.

3. Everyone needs the same nutrients, but in varying amounts.

   Elite athletes, recreational athletes, and sedentary people all require the same nutrients. But the amount of nutrients needed are influenced by age, sex, body size, level of activity, and state of health. As such, these factors must be considered when making nutritional recommendations to athletes.

What is the best diet for an athlete? This question still eludes us. The best diet is one that considers physiological, sociological, and psychological factors. It should also be based on the individual athlete's food preferences, food choices, and food likes. The ideal place to start is with current advice from health and nutrition experts.

A. DIETARY GUIDELINES FOR AMERICANS

In 1980, the U.S. Department of Agriculture and Health and Human Services (HHS), jointly established the Dietary Guidelines for Americans.[5] The guidelines represent current thinking in the field of nutrition and have become the cornerstone for federal policies and programs regarding food, nutrition, and health.[6] Since their introduction, the Dietary Guidelines were revised in 1985, 1990, and again in 1995 to include recent findings between diet and health.

The Dietary guidelines are seven basic principles for developing and maintaining a healthy diet. They emphasize balance, variety, and moderation in the diet and should serve as the nutrition foundation for athletes.

The 1995 guidelines are

- Eat a variety of foods.
- Balance the food you eat with physical activity. Maintain or improve your weight.
- Choose a diet with plenty of grain products, vegetables, and fruits.
- Choose a diet low in fat, saturated fat, and cholesterol.
- Choose a diet moderate in sugar.
- Choose a diet moderate in salt and sodium.
- If you drink alcoholic beverages, do so in moderation.

B. FOOD GUIDE PYRAMID

Although the guidelines are important when choosing foods for a healthier diet, they do not indicate how much of what foods to eat. The Food Guide Pyramid is one tool designed to help all individuals achieve a healthy diet.[7] Developed by the USDA and HHS in 1992, the Pyramid is an outline of what types of food and how much of each to eat everyday (Figure 2.1). Each of the five food groups provides essential nutrients; no one group is more important than another. For example, if the milk, yogurt, and cheese group are omitted, the best sources of calcium, riboflavin, and vitamin D are excluded from the diet. The tip of the pyramid represents fats, oils, and sweets. There is no serving size suggested for these products.

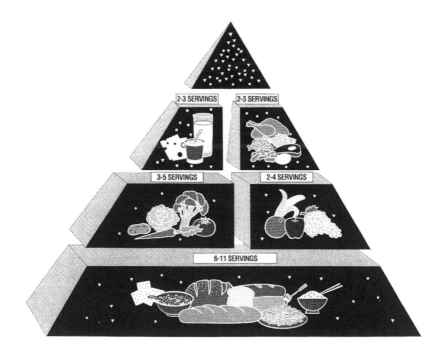

2-3 SERVINGS   2-3 SERVINGS

3-5 SERVINGS   2-4 SERVINGS

6-11 SERVINGS

FIGURE 2.1 The Food Guide Pyramid.

Each food group visually displays a range of servings which takes into account varying energy needs and personal food preferences. Everyone should eat the lowest number of servings to obtain an adequate supply of essential nutrients. The high end of the range is more appropriate for an endurance athlete consuming a high-carbohydrate, high-calorie diet. Figure 2.2 provides more information on how to use the Daily Food Guide.

Although the Dietary Guidelines and The Food Pyramid provide a standard by which individuals can measure the total diet, little has been done to assess the quality of the diet. In 1995, the USDA designed the Healthy Eating Index to provide a means of measuring eating habits of Americans. The

What counts as a serving?

Breads, cereals, rice, and pasta
1 slice of bread
½ cup of cooked rice or pasta
½ cup of cooked cereal
1 ounce of ready-to-eat cereal
2 cookies (medium)

Vegetables
½ cup cooked chopped raw or cooked vegetables
1 cup of leafy raw vegetables
3/4 cup vegetable juice

Fruits
1 piece of fruit or melon wedge
3/4 cup of juice
½ cup of canned fruit
1/4 cup of dried fruit

Milk, yogurt, and cheese
1 cup of milk or yogurt
1 ½ cups ice cream or ice milk
1 cup frozen yogurt

Meat, poultry, fish, dry beans, eggs, and nuts
2 ½ to 3 ounces of cooked lean meat,
 poultry, or fish
count ½ cup of cooked beans, or 1
egg, or 2 tablespoons of peanut butter
as 1 ounce of lean meat (about 1/3 serving)

Approximate number of servings needed each day

Calorie level	Lower 1,600	Moderate 2,200	High 2,800	Higher 3,600
Group				
Bread	6	9	11	14
Vegetable	3	4	5	7
Fruit	2	3	4	5
Milk	3	3	3	4
Meat (ounces)	5	6	7	9

FIGURE 2.2 How to use the daily food guide. Adapted from the *Food Guide Pyramid,* Home and Garden Bulletin Number 252, U.S. Department of Agriculture, Human Nutrition Information Service, 1992.

Healthy Eating Index (HEI) was developed based on a 10-component system of five food groups, four nutrients, and a measure of variety in food intake (Table 2.1).[8]

Although the Healthy Eating Index has not been tested specifically with athletes, it has been used to analyze a representative sample of the U.S. population.[8]

TABLE 2.1   Components of Healthy Eating Index

Food group	Range of scores	Perfect score of 10[a]
1. Grains	0 to 10	6 to 11 servings
2. Vegetables	0 to 10	3 to 5 servings
3. Fruits	0 to 10	2 to 4 servings
4. Milk	0 to 10	2 to 3 servings
5. Meat	0 to 10	2 to 3 servings
Dietary Guidelines		
6. Total fat	0 to 10	30% or less energy from fat
7. Saturated fat	0 to 10	Less than 10% energy from saturated fat
8. Cholesterol	0 to 10	300 mg or less
9. Sodium	0 to 10	2400 mg or less
10. Variety	0 to 10	16 different food items over 3-day period

[a] The number of recommended servings depends on an individual's caloric requirements.

From United States Department of Agriculture, *The Healthy Eating Index,* CNPP-1, 1995.

C. NUTRITION LABELING

As a result of the Nutrition Labeling and Education Act of 1990, food labels now include more information to help consumers make wise food choices. Nutrition labels are required on virtually all packaged goods and must conform with federal guidelines. According to law, every food label must state (1) the net content in terms of weight, measure, or count, and (2) the ingredients in descending order of predominance by weight.

Three of the important features found on food labels are "Nutrition Facts," descriptors, and health claims. The "Nutrition Facts" panel on most packaged food includes the serving size, number of servings per container, calories per servings and the number of calories from fat (Figure 2.3).

One of the most significant changes found on nutrition labels is the Daily Reference Value or Daily Value. Under the new guidelines, the Daily Value replaces the U.S. RDA, which was the old daily nutrient standard used on food labels. Daily Values appear for the nutrients that pose the greatest health risks, namely, total fat, saturated fat, cholesterol, sodium, carbohydrates, fiber, sugar, protein, vitamins A and C, and the minerals, iron and calcium. The Daily Values are based on a 2,000 calorie diet with 30% of the calories from fat (less than 20 g saturated), 60% from carbohydrates, and 10% from protein. This calculates to approximately 65 g of fat, 300 g of carbohydrates, 50 g of protein and 25 g of fiber. These labeling standards, established by the government, are based on current nutrition recommendations for health prevention. Thus, athletes' daily values may be higher due to higher calorie intakes and expenditures.

Serving sizes are more consistent across product lines, stated in both household and metric measures, and reflect the amounts people actually eat.

The list of nutrients covers those most important to the health of today's consumers, most of whom need to worry about getting too much of certain items (e.g. fat), rather than too few vitamins or minerals, as in the past.

The label also tells the number of calories per gram of fat, carbohydrates, and protein.

Calories from fat are shown on the label to help consumers meet dietary guidelines that recommend people get no more than 30 percent of their calories from fat.

% Daily Value shows how a food fits into the overall daily diet.

Daily values are relatively new. Some are maximums, as with fat (65 grams or less); others are minimums, as with carbohydrates (300 grams or more). The daily values on the label are based on a daily diet of 2,000 and 2,500 calories per day. Individuals should adjust the values to fit their own calorie intake.

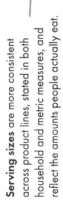

Nutrition Facts
Serving Size ½ cup (114g)
Servings Per Container 4

Amount Per Serving

Calories 90   Calories from Fat 30

	% Daily Value*
Total Fat 3g	5%
Saturated Fat 0g	0%
Cholesterol 0mg	0%
Sodium 300mg	13%
Total Carbohydrate 13g	4%
Dietary Fiber 3g	12%
Sugars 3g	
Protein 3g	

Vitamin A	80%	•	Vitamin C	60%
Calcium	4%	•	Iron	4%

* Percent Daily Values are based on a 2,000 calorie diet. Your daily values may be higher or lower depending on your calorie needs:

	Calories	2,000	2,500
Total Fat	Less than	65g	80g
Sat Fat	Less than	20g	25g
Cholesterol	Less than	300mg	300mg
Sodium	Less than	2,400mg	2,400mg
Total Carbohydrate		300g	375g
Fiber		25g	30g

Calories per gram:
Fat 9   •   Carbohydrates 4   •   Protein 4

FIGURE 2.3   Nutrition Facts label. (From The Food and Drug Administration.)

1. Common Terms Used on Food Labels

Descriptors are terms like "cholesterol-free" and "light" that describe a food's level of nutrients. Listed below are some common food label terms.

Sodium:
  Sodium free — less than 5 mg per serving
  Very low sodium — 35 mg or less per serving
  Low sodium — 140 mg or less per serving
Fat and cholesterol:
  Fat free — containing 0.5 g or less of fat per serving
  Low cholesterol — containing fewer than 20 mg of cholesterol per
    serving and fewer than 2 g saturated fat per serving
  Low fat — containing 3 g or less fat per serving
  Low saturated fat — containing 1 g or less saturated fat per serving

The Food and Drug Administration has established new definitions for the words *high*, *good source*, and *light* (or *lite*). A food containing 20% or more of the Daily Value is considered a "high," or excellent source of this nutrient. For example, yogurt is an excellent source of calcium because it contains 200 milligrams or more of calcium per serving. To be considered a "good" source of a particular nutrient, a food should provide 10 to 19% of that nutrient.

There is more than one approved definition for the term *light*. Products containing one third fewer calories or 50% less fat than the reference food can be labeled *light*. The term *light* is also used to describe texture or color, as in "light brown sugar."

2. Health Claims

Some food products carry health claims. A health claim is a statement that describes the relationship between a particular nutrient and disease, such as fat and heart disease. As of 1993, the FDA has approved seven claims linking nutrients and food to disease:

- Calcium and risk of osteoporosis
- Sodium and risk of high blood pressure
- Dietary fat and risk of cancer
- Dietary saturated fat and cholesterol and risk of coronary heart disease
- Fruits, vegetables, and grain products that contain fiber, particularly soluble fiber, and risk of coronary heart disease
- Fruits and vegetables and risk of cancer

These health claims are allowed on food labels because they are well supported by scientific studies. Thus, they are of great value to individuals who would rather not bother with grams, percentages, and other nutrient calculations.

III. DIETARY RECOMMENDATIONS FOR ATHLETES

Beyond healthy eating, athletes must meet nutrient needs for optimal performance. Athletes want to know what kinds of foods to eat, as well as specific dietary regimens to follow. Basically, the nutritional needs of athletes are similar to nonathletes, with the exception of calories and fluids. A diet that provides a variety of foods supplying 55 to 65% of calories as carbohydrates, 12 to 15% of calories as protein, and 20 to 30% of calories as fat is recommended for health and performance.[9] However, some types of heavy training increase the requirement for certain nutrients, such as carbohydrates and protein.

A. CARBOHYDRATES: THE ENERGY FOOD

Most athletes are aware of the importance of carbohydrates for optimal performance. However, they are often not as knowledgeable about the amounts and types of dietary carbohydrate needed during the various phases of training and competition. Additionally, athletes frequently are not aware of which foods are good carbohydrate sources.[10] For instance, female athletes may consider a large dinner salad a suitable high-carbohydrate meal. A basic knowledge of what carbohydrates are and their role in exercise will help the female athlete plan a diet that best meets her performance goals.

1. Characteristics and Functions

Carbohydrates are compounds containing mainly carbon, hydrogen, and oxygen. Sugars, starches, and fiber are the major forms in which carbohydrates occur in food. Starches and sugars are the body's main source of energy, supplying 4 kcal/g, while fiber provides bulk and aids in digestion.

Carbohydrates include both simple sugars and complex carbohydrates depending on the number of saccharide (sugar) units they contain. Simple sugars (glucose, fructose, and galactose) are monosaccharides, or single-saccharide units. They are the building blocks of more complex carbohydrates.

Glucose is the most common monosaccharide; it is the form of carbohydrate circulating in the blood. Glucose, fructose, and galactose are absorbed in the bloodstream, although fructose and galactose must be converted to glucose in the liver before entering the bloodstream.

The disaccharides (sucrose, lactose, and maltose) are composed of two simple sugar units joined together. Sucrose (table sugar) is the most common disaccharide; it is a combination of glucose and fructose. Lactose, sometimes referred to as milk sugar, is found only in milk products. It is composed of glucose and galactose. Maltose is a disaccharide composed of two glucose units. It appears whenever starch is being broken down.

Complex carbohydrates, also known as the polysaccharides, contain thousands of glucose units. Some of the most common polysaccharides of nutritional importance are starch, glycogen, and cellulose (fiber). Starches are found in whole grains, pasta, potatoes, legumes, and cereals. They are digested and absorbed into the bloodstream as glucose, which is the only carbohydrate form that can be used directly by the muscles for energy.

Glycogen is the storage form of glucose in the body. Two thirds of the glycogen in the body is stored in the muscles; the remaining one third is stored in the liver. The conversion of glucose to glycogen in the liver is a process called glycogenesis. The liver has the highest glycogen content of all the tissues in the body. In fact, it can convert many of the end-products of digestion (amino acids, fatty acids) into glycogen.

Cellulose (fiber) is found only in plant foods such as fruits, vegetables, and grains. Humans lack the enzyme necessary for its breakdown into simple sugars and for this reason fiber cannot be digested by the body.

The major function of fiber is to provide bulk or roughage which has important health benefits. Most high-fiber foods contain both soluble and insoluble fiber, but in different proportions. Insoluble fiber produces the tough, chewy texture of wheat bran, whole grains, and vegetables. Soluble fiber includes pectin and gum which is found in oats, dry beans and peas, and some fruits and vegetables. Eating foods containing insoluble fiber is important for proper bowel function and for reducing symptoms of chronic constipation, diverticulosis, and hemmorrhoids. Soluble fiber is said to help reduce blood cholesterol levels and control blood glucose levels in diabetics.

There is no RDA for fiber. The National Cancer Institute suggests consuming between 20 to 30 g/d of dietary fiber, which is about half the amount female athletes eat. Despite important health benefits, many athletes find high fiber intakes cause bloating, diarrhea, and gas. Too much fiber can limit food intake which can negatively affect energy balance. High-fiber diets can also interfere with the absorption of key nutrients such as iron, calcium, and zinc. Thus, female athletes should gradually increase fiber intake during training to determine what works best for them. Table 2.2 provides good souces of dietary fiber.

2. The Role of Carbohydrates In Exercise

The importance of carbohydrate as an energy substrate during exercise is well established. More than 30 years ago, scientists recognized three important facts. First, they recognized that depletion of carbohydrates in the form of glycogen is a limiting factor for exercise.[12] Second, they found that the amount of glycogen stored in muscle can be increased by consuming carbohydrate.[13] Third, they discovered that increased glycogen stores can enhance performance capacity.[14]

During exercise, muscles need energy to perform. The energy to perform work comes from the energy yielding nutrients — carbohydrates, protein, and fat. However, the muscles cannot directly use these nutrients for fuel. Instead, an energy-rich compound known as adenosine triphosphate (ATP) is the fuel for all energy-requiring processes. Muscles make and use ATP to do their

TABLE 2.2   Good Sources of Dietary Fiber

Food	Serving size	Fiber (g)
Refried beans	½ cup	11.0
Kelloggs All-Bran	1 oz	10.0
Pinto beans	½ cup	9.7
Kidney beans	½ cup	9.5
Almonds, dried	½ cup	8.7
Prunes, dried	10 each	8.0
Raspberries, fresh	1 cup	7.7
Peas, green, cooked fresh	1 cup	7.7
Strawberries, frozen	1 cup	7.6
Baked beans	½ cup	6.9
Pistachios, dried	½ cup	6.9
Squash, acorn	1 cup	6.9
Dates, pitted	10 each	6.8
Broccoli, cooked frozen	1 cup	5.4
Blueberries, frozen	1 cup	5.4

Note: Fiber is a plant material that cannot be digested by humans. It is found in beans and peas, fruits and vegetables, whole grains, and nuts. Fiber is important for proper bowel function and may help reduce the risk of heart disease and certain forms of cancer.

Health professionals recommend eating 20 to 30 g of dietary fiber daily.

work. However, muscles can store only a small amount of ATP, and it is depleted within the first few seconds of exercise. ATP is replenished by glycogen, the storage form of carbohydrate in the muscles and liver.

Unlike protein and fat, carbohydrate stores in the body are limited. When glycogen levels are low or depleted, the ability to exercise at a relatively high intensity (65–85% VO_{2max}) is impaired.[13] The athlete who does not consume enough calories will have difficulty meeting carbohydrate requirements. As a result, performance can suffer due to fatigue and reduced exercise capacity.

Consuming adequate carbohydrates serves to maintain blood glucose levels and to keep glycogen stores in the muscles from being depleted.[15] Carbohydrates also provide a protein sparing effect. The body uses carbohydrates as a source of energy when it is provided in the diet. This allows protein to be "saved" for building and repairing body tissues.

3. How Much Carbohydrate Do Athletes Need?

Carbohydrate requirements vary depending on age and body size. An athlete with more muscle mass will require more carbohydrate. The amount of carbohdyrates needed also depends on the intensity and level of training. Endurance athletes who train aerobically for more than 90 min daily need approximately 8 to 10 grams of carbohydrate/kg bw/d to adequately restore glycogen levels.[15] This amount is equivalent to 560 to 700 total grams of carbohydrate or 60 to 70% of total calorie intake. Many female endurance athletes have difficulty achieving this level. Studies[16-18] show that few female athletes consume more than 6 g/kg bw/d of carbohydrates. The carbohydrate content of selected foods is shown in Table 2.3.

Determining the carbohydrate requirements of nonendurance athletes has been difficult because most of the research proposing that athletes eat a high-carbohydrate diet has been conducted on endurance athletes such as runners and cyclists. The majority of athletes, however, participate in sports like gymnastics, ballet, figure skating, and team sports such as basketball, volley-ball, tennis, and track. These sports generally involve brief periods of high-intensity exercise with alternate rest periods and may not reduce muscle glycogen to the same degree as continuous exercise for the same amount of time.

Research shows that glycogen availability is not a limiting factor during a single, brief bout of exercise of maximal intensity.[19] However, high-intensity, intermittent activity can reduce muscle glycogen to critically low levels and impair performance.[20] Soccer players, for example, are required to exercise continually at high intensities using large muscle groups for periods of several seconds to several minutes throughout a game.[21] Muscle glycogen concentration decreases in proportion to the duration and intensity of the game depending on the level of competition, how well trained the athlete is, and initial body carbohydrate stores.[21]

Jacobs et al.[22] studied the effects of dietary repletion patterns on muscle glycogen levels in elite soccer players after a regular game and for two days thereafter. Muscle glycogen levels were low (45.9 ± 7.9 mmol glucose units) following the game, and after 48 hours had increased only to 72.8 mmol glucose units. The authors attributed the players' inability to maintain normal glycogen levels to their eating habits. Diet records revealed that the players consumed only an average of 47% of their calories from carbohydrates, whereas 60 to 65% is recommended.[15]

It is possible that the nonendurance athlete who trains daily and consumes a low-carbohydrate diet is at risk for reduced muscle glycogen levels that could impair training and performance. Thus, eating adequate carbohydrates is essential to maintaining muscle glycogen levels during training and workouts. This may be even more important for the nonendurance athlete who is restricting calories to maintain a low body weight.

B. CARBOHYDRATES BEFORE, DURING, AND AFTER EXERCISE

Because carbohydrates are a vital energy substrate for muscles during prolonged strenuous exercise, nutritional strategies to increase glycogen stores before, during, and after exercise are imperative. This section will discuss briefly the specific carbohydrate needs for endurance training and competition.

TABLE 2.3   Carbohydrate Content of Selected Foods

Foods	Amount	Carbohydrate (g)	Foods	Amount	Carbohydrate (g)
Fruits			Popcorn, plain	1/2 c	2
Apple (whole)	1	21	Pretzels	4	19
Apple juice	1/2 c	15	Rice, brown	1/2 c	23
Apple (dried)	1/2 c	28	Rice, white	1/2 c	17
Apricot (dried)	1/2 c	40	Tortilla (flour)	1	17
Banana (dried)	1	27	Whole wheat	1 slice	13
Cantaloupe	1/2 c	7	bread		
Cranberry juice	1/2 c	19	Milk products		
Fig (whole)	1	10	1% milk	1 c	12
Grapes	1/2 c	8	2% milk	1 c	12
Grape juice	1/2 c	19	Skim milk	1 c	12
Orange (whole)	1	15	Pudding	1 c	63
Orange juice	1/2 c	12	Yogurt, frozen	1 c	42
Peach (whole)	1	10	Yogurt, fruit	1 c	43
Peaches	1/2 c	7	flavored		
Pear (whole)	1	30	Yogurt, plain	1 c	16
Pears	1/2 c	9	Sugars		
Pineapple	1/2 c	10	Candy		
Raisins	1/2 c	57	Granola bars	1	16
Watermelon	1/2 c	6	Gum drops	1 oz	25
Vegetables			Cookies		
Carrots	1/2 c	8	Chocolate	1	7
Corn	1/2 c	17	chip		
Peas (sweet)	1/2 c	11	Fig bars	1	11
Potatoes (white)	1/2 c	16	Oatmeal/raisin	1	8
Sweet potato	1/2 c	33	Jam	1 T	14
Tomato, fresh	1/2 c	3	Jelly	1 T	13
Tomato juice	1/2 c	5	Soft drinks	1 c	25
Grains/legumes			Commercial sports		
Angel food cake	1 slice	32	drinks/foods		
Bagel	1	31	Gatorade®	1 c	15
Bun	1	20	GatorLode®	1 c	47
Bran muffin	1	17	GatorPro®	1 c	58
Cereals			Exceed®-fluid	1 c	17
Cheerios	1/2 c	8	replacement		
Oatmeal	1/2 c	13	Exceed®-high carb.	1 c	59
Shredded	1 biscuit	18	Exceed®-sports	1 c	54
wheat			meal		
Crackers			Nutrament®	1 c	30
Graham	1	5	Power Bar®	1	40
Saltines	1	2	Combinations		
Rye Krisp	1	5	Chicken noodle	1 c	9
Rice cake	1	8	soup		
English muffin	1	26	Macaroni and	1/2 c	13
Garbanzo beans	1/3 c	10	cheese		
Kidney beans	1/3 c	13	Pizza, cheese	1 slice	16
Pancakes	1	9	Potato salad	1/2 c	14
Pasta	1/2 c	15	Spaghetti	1 c	33
Pita bread	1 slice	21	w/tomato sauce		

TABLE 2.3 (continued)   Carbohydrate Content of Selected Foods

Foods	Amount	Carbohydrate (g)	Foods	Amount	Carbohydrate (g)
Taco, meat	1	27	Split Pea soup	1 c	28
Tomato soup	1 c	17	Vegetable soup	1 c	12

From Houtkooper, L., Food selection for endurance sports. *Med. Sci. Sports. Exerc.* 24, S349–S359, 1992. With permission.

1. Before Exercise

Research has shown that athletes who consume carbohydrates before exercise have the potential to significantly increase their carbohydrate stores and enhance training and performance capacity.[23] In a study by Sherman et al.,[24] cycling performance was improved by 15% when athletes consumed 312 g of liquid carbohydrate (4.5 g/kg bw) 4 hours before moderately intense exercise. Consuming from 1 to 4.5 g of carbohydrate/kg from one to 4 hours before exercise will help maintain blood glucose levels during exercise and ensure adequate carbohydrate availability.[23,24] Athletes who fast prior to competition risk decreasing their blood glucose levels during exercise and impaired performance.

2. Glycemic Index

At one time, it was believed that simple sugars (glucose, fructose) were digested and absorbed quickly, causing a rapid rise in blood glucose levels. It was also assumed that complex carbohdyrates were digested at a much slower rate, providing a small increase in blood glucose levels. What we now know is that the effect of carbohydrates on blood glucose is dependent on many factors including the form of food, its digestibility, how it is cooked, and whether it is eaten alone or as part of a mixed meal.

The glycemic index is a rating scale used to determine how fast or completely a carbohydrate food is digested and absorbed in the blood stream.[25] Foods with a high glycemic index (>85) provide a quick rise in blood glucose levels whereas low glycemic foods (<60) supply long-term sustained energy (Table 2.4). The higher the index number, the quicker a food may raise blood glucose levels. Because glucose causes more of a blood-sugar response than any other food, it has a value of 100. Note that "simple" and "complex" carbohydrates are not synonymous with "high" and "low" glycemic foods on the index scale. One might assume that complex carbohydrates would have a low glycemic index rating, but this is not always the case. Cooked carrots, for example, have a glycemic index of 92, which is almost as high as glucose. Differences among complex carbohydrates also exist. Horowitz and Coyle[26] observed the glycemic response to various meals with the same carbohydrate content before exercise and found the glycemic response to potato to be significantly greater than that for rice.

TABLE 2.4   Glycemic Index of Selected Foods

High (over 80)	Medium (60 to 80)	Low (less than 60)
Glucose	Bread, whole wheat	Spaghetti
Cornflakes	Rice, white	Sweet corn
Potatoes, instant	Broad beans	Sucrose
Carrots, cooked	Potato, new	All-Bran
Parsnips	Shredded Wheat	Potato chips
Maltose	Bananas	Oranges
Honey	Raisins	Orange juice
	Mars candy bar	Apples
	Rice, brown	Tomato soup
		Ice cream
		Milk
		Yogurt
		Beans, kidney
		Peanuts

Adapted from Jenkins, D.J.A., et al., Glycemic Index of Foods: a physiological basis for carbohydrate exchange. *Am. J. Clin. Nutr.,* 34, 362–366, 1981. With permission.

Research shows that low glycemic-index foods are advantageous before exercise because they provide a slow-release source of glucose to the blood without an accompanying surge of insulin.[27] Thomas et al.[27] observed the effect of foods of differing glycemic index on athletes and their performance during exercise. Eight trained cyclists pedaled to exhaustion 1 hour after consuming a test meal of either lentils, potato, glucose, or water. Endurance time was significantly longer in the lentils trial than the potato, glucose, or water trials. Results of this preliminary study indicate that low glycemic foods may be optimal prior to exercise.

3. During Exercise

Consuming carbohydrates during exercise can delay fatigue and improve performance by preventing blood glucose levels from declining in the latter stages of prolonged exercise.[28,29] Findings by Wright et al.[30] showed that consuming 0.2 g carbohydrate/kg bw every 20 min resulted in a 32% improvement in endurance time and a 34% improvement in total work output.

Although carbohydrate consumption during exercise can delay fatigue, it cannot prevent it. Carbohydrates offer the greatest benefit during prolonged exercise that is limited by carbohydrate availability.[31] The optimal time to consume carbohydrate is during the latter stages of prolonged exercise (e.g., 30 min prior to the point of fatigue) when muscle glycogen and blood glucose levels are low.[32]

Which are better during exercise, solid or liquid carbohydrates? Lugo et al.[33] examined the effects of consuming a 7% carbohydrate-electrolyte beverage and 0.4 g carbohydrate/kg bw/d in the form of a sport bar immediately before and every 30 min during 120 min of cycling at 70% VO_{2max}. Results showed that carbohydrate availability was similar for both. Ultimately, the type of carbohydrate used during exercise should be determined by what is best tolerated under performance conditions.[34] Both liquids and solids offer different advantages for the athlete.[35] Liquids are easier to consume than solids during exercise and also provide fluid replacement.[34] Solid foods offer substance and are convenient for athletes in sports such as cycling, swimming, and skiing. Athletes should experiment with different types of carbohydrates during training to determine what works best.

How much carbohydrate should athletes consume during exercise? Coyle[34] concludes that 30 to 60 g/h in the form of solutions containing glucose, sucrose, or maltodextrins will help maintain blood glucose levels during exercise and enhance endurance capacity.

4. After Exercise: The Recovery Period

The timing and amount of carbohydrates consumed after exercise is critical, particularly for athletes competing in multiple events on a single day or several days in a row. The sooner athletes eat after exercise, the faster their recovery rate of muscle glycogen.[36] It is best to eat carbohydrates immediately after exercise; delaying carbohydrate consumption for even 2 hours after exercise can reduce the rate at which carbohydrates are used by the body by 50%.[36]

Endurance athletes should consume at least 1.5 g of carbohydrate/kg bw immediately and again 2 hours after exercise to maximize glycogen resynthesis.[37] For a 130 lb (59 kg) female athlete, this would amount to approximately 89 g of carbohydrate. If the athlete weighs less or if the level of exercise is not as intense, carbohydrate requirements will be lower.

Does the type of carbohydrate consumed affect the rate of muscle glycogen storage? Reed et al.[38] demonstrated that consumption of either solid or liquid carbohydrate produced similar rates of muscle glycogen synthesis. In another study, Blom et al.[39] showed that the rate of muscle glycogen synthesis was similar for glucose or sucrose, but 50% lower with fructose. Athletes can restore muscle glycogen by consuming either liquid (sport drinks, juices) or solid carbohydrate. Eating a combination of the two, however, may be the most practical approach. Tanaka et al.[16] reported that following exercise, female distance runners consumed solids (i.e., dry cereal and breads) more than liquids, and glucose more than fructose or sucrose.

Carbohydrates with a moderate to high glycemic index should take priority in the recovery diet. Results by Burke et al.[40] showed that consuming high glycemic carbohydrate foods after prolonged exercise produced significantly greater glycogen storage than did low glycemic foods.

5. Carbohydrate Loading

Carbohydrate loading is the process of manipulating the diet and amount of exercise in an attempt to increase glycogen stores in the muscles. There are several variations of carbohydrate loading. The most effective regimen with the fewest side effects is one developed by Sherman and Costill.[41] They recommend three days of a mixed diet followed by three days of a high-carbohydrate diet in concert with depletion-tapering exercise the week before competition and complete rest the day before the event. The diet should provide adequate calories and 500 to 600 g/d of carbohydrate or >8 g/kg bw/d. This regimen should increase muscle glycogen stores ≥20 to 40% above normal.[34]

Carbohydrate loading can easily be accomplished with foods and beverages, provided the athlete has a basic knowledge of the amounts and types of carbohydrates. According to Burke and Read,[42] without specific instructions or knowledge of nutrition and food composition, athletes may be limited in their ability to achieve the dietary requirements of carbohydrate loading. In their survey of marathon runners, the average amount of carbohydrates consumed on "loading" days was 469 g, with individual intakes ranging from 188 to 960 g. This represents an average of 53% of total energy intake.

Tarnopolsky et al.[43] demonstrated that female athletes do not increase muscle glycogen levels in response to carbohydrate loading to the same degree as male athletes. They fed a high-carbohydrate diet (75% of energy from carbohydrates) or low carbohydrate diet (55 to 60% of energy) to 7 male and 8 female athletes over a four day period. Additionally, they examined whether gender differences existed in metabolism during submaximal endurance cycling at 75% VO_{2max}. Results showed that the men increased muscle glycogen concentrations by 41% in response to carbohydrate loading and had a corresponding increase in performance time. The women, however, did not increase glycogen levels or performance time. Tarnopolsky et al.[43] offers three possible explanations for gender differences:

1. The higher muscle glycogen response to carbohydrate in men may be due in part to a greater post-exercise glycogen depletion.
2. Female athletes, because they are smaller in body size and consume fewer calories than men, may not be able to achieve the level of carbohydrate needed to "load."
3. The phase of the menstrual cycle is an important consideration for female athletes. During the luteal phase of the menstrual cycle, progesterone levels are higher which may reverse the increased use of fats and decreased carbohydrate oxidation.

Tarnopolsky and colleagues[43] summarized by saying that knowledge of these gender differences is important because dietary recommendations based on studies involving primarily male subjects may not be appropriate for women. Thus, their study emphasizes the need for more gender-specific, sport-specific nutrition recommendations.

Carbohydrate loading is advantageous for endurance athletes but it is not shown to be beneficial for athletes participating in nonendurance sports. Potential side effects of carbohydrate loading include increased water retention and subsequent weight gain. Stiffness and a feeling of heaviness have also been reported. Furthermore, some athletes may experience stomach upset (flatulence and diarrhea) on very high-carbohdyrate diets.

C. PROTEIN
1. Characteristics and Functions

Proteins are complex organic compounds containing the elements carbon, hydrogen, oxygen, nitrogen, and sometimes sulfur. They are necessary for growth, the building of new tissue, and for repairing injured tissue. The skin, tendons, and contractile elements in muscles are made of proteins. All enzymes and most hormones, such as epinephrine and insulin, are composed of protein. Protein also serves as a potential source of energy, with each gram providing approximately 4 kcal. The body's energy requirements, however, must be satisfied before it can efficiently use proteins for growth and repair. This means if the diet does not provide sufficient calories from carbohydrates and fat, protein will be broken down and used for energy instead of being used for building and repairing tissue.

Just as monosaccharides are the building blocks of carbohydrates, amino acids are the basic units of protein. At present, 20 different amino acids have been identified. Amino acids differ in their individual characteristics; some are sweet, some are sour, and some are bitter. They also differ in the way that they are supplied to the body.

Amino acids are needed for growth and repair of body cells and tissues. Some amino acids are nonessential, meaning they can be made in the body if an adequate source of nitrogen (other amino acids) is available. The others are known as essential amino acids; they cannot be synthesized in the body and must be supplied from food. The essential amino acids for humans are isoleucine, leucine, lysine, methionine, threonine, phenylalanine, tryptophan, valine, and histidine.

The quality of dietary protein needed to promote growth depends on many factors, such as the presence of essential amino acids in the right quantity and proportion, an adequate intake of the nonessential amino acids, and an adequate intake of calories.[44] Good quality protein supplies a mixture of amino acids in proportions similar to our own tissue proteins.

Proteins that contain all the amino acids (essential and nonessential) have a high biological value and are known as complete proteins. They are found in animal sources such as meat, fish, dairy products, and eggs. In comparison, many plant proteins are low in specific amino acids. For example, lysine is consistently lower in all plant food groups (legumes, nuts and seeds, cereals, and fruits) than in animal foods.[44] The sulfur-containing amino acids are lower in cereals and legumes but higher in nuts and seeds than animal foods.[44] Therefore, consuming mixtures of plant proteins will provide for an adequate protein intake.[45]

2. The Role of Protein In Exercise

Although protein does not serve as a major source of energy during exercise, research shows that both endurance and strength training increase the need for protein in the diet.[46] This increased need may occur directly, as a result of changes in amino acid metabolism, or indirectly, as a result of insufficient energy intake.[47] Studies[48,49] show that exercise causes an increased utilization of several amino acids, particularly the branched-chain amino acids (leucine, isoleucine, and valine), and that under certain conditions, such as decreased muscle glycogen,[50] total oxidation may become significant.

The metabolism of protein during exercise depends upon several factors including the type, intensity, and duration of exercise, carbohydrate intake, energy intake, age, and gender.[51] To assess changes in protein metabolism, nutritionists often use a measurement known as nitrogen balance. Nitrogen is a major component of protein. By measuring the amount of nitrogen excreted by the body (i.e., urine, feces, and sweat), one can tell how protein is being used. A positive nitrogen balance means that the athlete is consuming enough protein and the body is using that protein to build muscle tissue. However, when protein intake is not adequate, a negative nitrogen balance can occur. In this case, the body is using its own protein stores for energy instead of building and repairing body tissues.

A negative nitrogen balance can result if the athlete is not eating enough protein. It can also occur if the athlete is not consuming enough calories. Energy is the body's first priority. Protein requirements increase when calorie intake is low. This is one reason why protein intake is a concern among female athletes, because many do not consume enough calories or they limit their intake of meat, poultry, fish, and dairy products, which are good sources of protein.

3. Protein Requirements of Endurance Athletes

Although the RDA of 0.8 g/kg of protein may be sufficient for individuals who do aerobic-type exercise at a relatively low intensity,[52] as the intensity of exercise increases, so will protein requirements, especially if the athlete is not consuming enough calories. Based on nitrogen balance studies,[53-56] endurance athletes require between 1.2 and 1.4 g/kg bw/d of protein. This additional protein is needed to cover for the increased loss of amino acids during exercise and to help repair exercise-induced muscle damage.[46] However, as indicated by Lemon[46] in his review on protein and amino acids, many of the studies conducted on protein requirements of endurance athletes have been obtained on male athletes. Preliminary data suggest that there may be differences in the protein requirements of male and female athletes.

Tarnopolsky et al.[57] studied gender differences in substrate utilization during exercise and reported higher carbohydrate and fat utilization in females, and possibly a greater protein utilization in males. In another study, Phillips et al.[58] examined nitrogen balance and leucine oxidation during submaximal endurance exercise in male and female endurance athletes, and they reported that male athletes oxidized more leucine during exercise than did females. For the women, a greater proportion of energy was obtained from fat. Thus, male athletes may have a higher protein requirement than female athletes.

4. Protein Requirements of Strength Athletes

Strength athletes often believe they need more protein to promote and maintain lean body mass. This is because protein is the nutrient most often associated with strength and physical performance. For centuries, athletes believed that to add muscle they needed to eat muscle. Milo of Croton, an Olympic heavyweight wrestler, was thought to consume a daily diet consisting of 20 lb of meat, 20 lb of bread, and 18 pints of wine.[59] However, if historical records are correct, the first athlete to train on a meat diet was Dromeus of Stymphalus, a long-distance runner of 480 BC.[59]

Although strength training can be very intense, the duration of exercise is short, and protein is not the most important energy source. Many athletes do not understand the dietary requirements for muscle gain. One pound of muscle is approximately 75% water, 20% protein, and 5% other materials such as fat, glycogen, minerals, and enzymes.[60] Thus, 1 lb of muscle equals about 105 g of protein. To gain one lb of muscle in 2 weeks, an athlete would need to consume 8 g of additional protein/d, this is equivalent to 1 oz of meat or cheese, an 8-oz glass of milk, or 4 slices of bread.

Although the protein requirements of strength athletes are still being studied, a review of the literature to date indicates a protein need of somewhere between 1.4 to 1.8 g/kg/d, depending on the type and intensity of training.[46] This is also assuming that the diet provides adequate calories and high-quality protein.

What about strength athletes who include aerobic exercise as part of their training program? Are their protein requirements greater? One would assume so, although research is limited. Increased protein intake may be necessary when athletes begin a training program or increase their training intensity.[61] However, as training continues and adaptation occurs, dependence upon a higher protein intake will decrease as long as adequate calories are consumed.

Reports indicate that some athletes, such as ballet dancers, female cyclists, distance runners, and bodybuilders limit their intake of red meat and adopt more vegetarian-like eating habits.[62-65] Barr[66] assessed the dietary patterns of Canadian female recreational athletes and found that 37% of the subjects classified themselves as "semivegetarian," excluding red meat from their diet. Slavin et al.[67] reported that one third of the female cyclists in their study (including recreational and elite racers) described their diets as vegetarian.

Although many athletes eat more protein than they need, female athletes may not be getting enough quality protein especially if they are restricting calories to maintain low body weight and consuming vegetarian diets.

5. Vegetarian Diets

Today the word *vegetarian* is a general term, since many types of vegetarian diets exist. They range from vegan, which excludes all animal products, to semivegetarian, which includes some groups of animal products (Table 2.5). Vegetarian eating habits are widespread in the world for both religious, moral, and economic reasons. In the U.S., people choose a vegetarian diet primarily for health reasons.[68] Vegetarians often make a commitment to a certain type of lifestyle that includes greater health awareness, i.e., reducing cholesterol levels, eating less fat, and avoiding alcohol and tobacco.[69]

TABLE 2.5   Glossary of Vegetarian Terms

Term	Definition
Vegan or Pure Vegetarian	Plant-food diet without any animal foods, milk products, or eggs.
Lacto Vegetarian	Plant-food diet supplemented with milk and milk products.
Lacto-ovo Vegetarian	Plant-food diet supplemented with eggs, milk, and milk products.
Semivegetarian	Plant-food diet supplemented with some groups of animal products.
New Vegetarian	Plant-food diet supplemented with some groups of animal products, but emphasis is placed on foods that are "organic," "natural," and unprocessed or unrefined.
Pescovegetarian	Excludes red meats, but consumes fish as well as plant foods.
Fruitarian	Diet consists of raw or dried fruits, nuts, seeds, honey, and vegetable oil.
Macrobiotic	Avoids all animal foods. Uses only unprocessed, unrefined, "natural" and "organic" foods. In some types, there is fluid restriction. Tamari, miso, and various seaweeds are used.

From Ruud, J.S. Vegetarianism—Implications for Athletes. *International Center for Sports Nutrition,* 1990.

For athletes consuming vegetarian diets, protein requirements may be slightly higher because of the lower quality of plant proteins. As previously mentioned, many vegetables and whole grains are low in specific amino acids. For example, cereals are low in the essential amino acid lysine. Legumes are low in the amino acid methionine. However, the quality of protein depends on the source and dietary mixture of plant protein. Thus, mixtures of plant proteins can be equivalent to animal proteins.

A bigger protein problem for athletes with vegetarian eating habits is quantity. Because vegetarian diets are higher in fibrous foods (fruits, vegetables, and grains), they also tend to be very filling. Thus, athletes consuming vegetarian diets may feel satisfied on fewer calories. When insufficient calories are consumed, more dietary protein is needed to maintain nitrogen balance. Lacto-ovo-vegetarian diets (plant-food diet supplemented with dairy foods and eggs) generally supply adequate calories and usable protein. However, athletes consuming pure vegan diets (plant-food diet with no aminal foods of any type) may have difficulty meeting energy and protein needs. Vegan diets should include tofu or other soy-based products. Research shows that well-processed soy-protein isolates and soy-protein concentrates can serve as the major source of dietary protein and that their protein value is equivalent to that of animal proteins.[70]

On the plus side, vegetarian diets supply a generous amount of complex carbohydrates, which go a long way toward sparing protein for building and repairing muscle tissue. Studies of vegetarians have reported mean carbohydrate intakes ranging from 45% of total calories for lacto-ovo-vegetarians,[71] to 60% for vegans.[72]

D. FATS

Today, many female athletes have become overly concerned about fat, both in their diets and on their bodies. The message that a high-fat diet contributes to obesity and the risk of chronic disease has affected female athletes eating habits and attitudes. Counting fat grams has become somewhat of an obsession. For many athletes the word "fat" signifies "weight."

It's true that too much fat either in the diet or on the body is not good for both health and performance reasons. But that is not where the story ends. There is another side to fat.

1. Characteristics and Functions

Fat serves several physiological functions in the body. It is the most concentrated source of energy, supplying twice as many calories (9 kcal/g) as either carbohydrates or protein. The subcutaneous layer of fat just beneath the skin insulates the body from heat loss. It also provides additional padding that protects vital organs, including the kidneys, heart, and liver, from injury.

Fat provides palatability to the diet and is responsible for the characteristic flavor, aroma, and texture of many foods. Foods containing fat stay in the stomach longer and digest at a slower rate, thus promoting satiety.

Fat functions as a carrier for the fat-soluble vitamins A, D, E, and K, and it supplies the body with the essential fatty acids linoleic acid and linolenic acid. These two polyunsaturated fatty acids cannot be made by the body and must be supplied by the diet. One tablespoon (14.8 ml) of polyunsaturated vegetable oil in salads, margarine, or other foods in a normal diet is enough to satisfy an adult's daily requirement.

Not all fats are alike and a general understanding of their characteristics can help define their role in health and performance.

Glycerides are the most common form of fat, consisting of one, two, or three fatty acids attached to a molecule of glycerol. The majority of glycerides found in food and in the body are triglycerides.

Fats are classified into three groups: saturated fat, monounsaturated fat, and polyunsaturated fat, based on their degree of saturation and carbon-chain length. Saturated fats are usually solid at room temperature. They are derived mainly from animal foods such as meat, poultry, and whole milk, but are also found in some vegetable products such as coconut oil, palm oil, and palm kernel oil. A diet high in saturated fat can raise blood cholesterol levels and increase the risk of heart disease and some cancers in certain individuals.

Monounsaturated fats are found mainly in vegetable oils and are usually liquid at room temperature. Examples include olive oil, safflower oil, and canola oil. Monounsaturated fats are reportedly the more healthful fats. They are associated with reduced blood cholesterol levels and a lower risk of heart disease.[73]

Polyunsaturated fats are found primarily in plant sources such as sunflower, corn, soybean, and safflower. They supply the body's need for essential fatty acids such as linoleic acid and linolenic acid. Polyunsaturated fats such as corn oil can help reduce high blood cholesterol levels.

2. Cholesterol

Cholesterol is an important structural and functional component of cell membranes. It is necessary for the production of bile (an emulsifier), vitamin D, and several hormones, including estrogen, androgen, and progesterone. Cholesterol is synthesized in the liver and intestine, and therefore is not considered essential in the diet. Dietary cholesterol is found in animal products such as meat, poultry, milk, and eggs. The body needs some cholesterol for good health, but it can make enough on its own.

Fat and cholesterol are transported in the bloodstream by lipoproteins, compounds formed when proteins combine with lipids. There are three major classes of lipoproteins in the blood: the chylomicrons, low-density lipoproteins, and high-density lipoproteins. High levels of low-density lipoproteins (LDL) are strongly associated with risk of heart disease.[73] Reducing saturated fat and cholesterol in the diet helps lower LDL-cholesterol levels in the blood.

High levels of high-density lipoproteins (HDL) appear to have a protective effect against heart disease. An individual's HDL levels can be increased with physical activity.[74]

3. The Role of Fat In Exercise

Both carbohydrates and fats contribute to energy metabolism during exercise. However, as previously stated, carbohydrates are the primary fuel for high-intensity exercise. At intensities of 70 to 80% VO_{2max} virtually all the glycogen in the muscles can be used within 1 to 2 hours.[14] In comparison, there is practically an unlimited supply of fat in the body, enough for several hours of low-intensity exercise.

The major advantage attributed to the use of fats as a source of energy during exercise is the role of fatty acid oxidation in sparing muscle glycogen.[75,76] During endurance exercise, carbohydrate reserves are depleted and the body relies on the breakdown of fat for energy production. When carbohydrate stores are low, the breakdown of fat ensures that the muscles' energy needs can be met. The ability to obtain a substantial proportion of energy from fat is important for athletes such as cyclists, runners, and triathletes who exercise for prolonged periods of time and need to conserve muscle glycogen stores for the latter stages of training or competition.

What factors control the amount of fat used during exercise? Basically, fat is controlled by the same factors that affect carbohydrates and protein: the intensity and duration of exercise, prior training, and diet.[77] Aerobic exercise promotes fat oxidation, whereas anaerobic exercise favors carbohydrate oxidation.[78] Furthermore, trained individuals oxidize more fat and fewer carbohydrates than nontrained subjects when exercising at the same intensity. Jansson and Kaijser[79] compared substrate utilization in the muscles of untrained subjects and endurance-trained competitive cyclists during exercise at the same intensity (65% VO_{2max}) and found that trained subjects oxidized more fat in relation to carbohydrates than untrained subjects. As mentioned previously, data also suggest that female athletes derive a greater proportion of their energy during exercise from fat in relation to carbohydrate or protein.[57,58] According to Ruby and Robergs,[80] the hormones regulating the menstrual cycle dramatically influence substrate selection and most likely account for gender differences.

4. How Much Dietary Fat Should Athletes Consume?

In 1990, the U.S. Department of Health and Human Services (DHHS) published *Healthy People 2000*, a set of health objectives for Americans to be reached by the year 2000.[81] The objectives are organized into 22 priority areas with 300 primary objectives, 21 of which are on nutrition.[82] (Table 2.6) Many of the nutrition objectives are consistent with the Dietary Guidelines for Americans and are aimed at reducing coronary heart disease, the risk of cancer, and the prevalence of obesity by targeting specific dietary changes.

TABLE 2.6   Healthy People 2000: Nutrition Objectives

Nutrient and Food Objectives

1. Reduce dietary fat intake
2. Increase intakes of complex carbohydrates and fiber-containing foods
3. Increase the proportion of overweight people taking effective steps to control their weight
4. Increase calcium intakes among teenagers, pregnant women, women who are breastfeeding their infants, and adults in general
5. Reduce salt intakes and purchases of foods high in salt
6. Remedy iron deficiencies in children and women
7. Encourage breastfeeding of infants immediately after birth and the continuation of breastfeeding for at least six months after birth
8. Teach parents infant-feeding practices that will minimize the chances of tooth decay

From *Healthy People 2000: National Health Promotion and Disease Prevention Objectives,* Washington, D.C., U.S. Department of Health and Human Services, 1990.

One of the nutrition objectives is to reduce dietary fat intake to an average of 30% of calories or less and saturated fat intake to less than 10% of calories. This objective is based on evidence showing a strong relationship between saturated fat intake, high blood cholesterol, and increased risk for heart disease.[83] Epidemiological studies also suggest that dietary fat can influence the risk of some cancers, particularly breast and colon cancer.[84] Furthermore, diets high in fat are associated with higher prevalences of overweight.[85]

Currently, there is no recommended dietary allowance for fat. Most heath experts suggest that athletes consume around 30% of total calories from fat. However, fat intakes will vary depending on the athlete's health, current eating habits, and performance goals. Obviously, female athletes with a family history of heart disease, cancer, or obesity should follow a low-fat diet for disease prevention. However, among healthy athletes, fat intakes can be slightly higher and not affect health and performance. Many athletes need a certain amount of calories from fat to meet energy requirements. In a review on the nutritional practices of elite athletes, total fat intake for female athletes ranged from 26 to 38% for endurance sports and 28 to 38% for nonendurance sports.[17] In comparison, the average American female consumes about 34% of calories from fat.[86]

The main disadvantage of a high fat diet for athletes is the dependence on fatty acids as the primary energy source, which can reduce the duration and capacity of exercise.[87] Thus, from a performance perspective, eating fat at the expense of carbohydrate is not recommended.[88]

While it is true that consuming too much fat is undesirable, having extremely low fat intakes is also unhealthy. Athletes who consume too little fat can suffer problems: low energy levels, menstrual irregularities, and inadequate nutrition. Decreased fat and energy intakes often lead to exclusion of foods such as red meat and dairy products. Keith et al.[63] reported that female cyclists consuming an average of 1781 kcal/d and 26% of calories from fat had low dietary intakes of several nutrients including iron, zinc, and vitamin B_6. Meats, poultry, fish, nuts, and peas were foods that were frequently omitted from the diet.

To determine approximately how many grams of fat an athlete should eat, multiply the number of calories per day by 0.30 (30%) to get the total calories from fat. Then divide the calories from fat by 9 (the number of kcal/g of fat) to get the total amount of fat/d. For example, for a female athlete who consumes 2400 kcal/d, 80 g of fat represents 30% of total calorie intake. Figure 2.4 shows how to calculate the grams of fat for different calorie levels.

IV. CONCLUSIONS

The best diet for an athlete is based on individual food preferences, food choices, and food likes. Most experts support The Dietary Guidelines for Americans and the Food Guide Pyramid as the foundation for a healthy diet.

Beyond healthy eating, athletes must meet nutrient needs for optimal performance. A balanced diet providing approximately 1.0 to 2.0 g of protein/kg bw/d, 6 to 8 g carbohydrate/kg bw/d, and 30% of total calories from fat is recommended for athletes. Because carbohydrates are a vital energy substrate for muscles during training and competition, nutritional strategies to increase glycogen stores before, during, and after exercise are imperative.

On the average, female athletes consume about 32 percent of total calories from fat. The Dietary Guidelines suggest a goal of 30 percent of total calories from fat. However, some athletes may need slightly more or less than this amount, depending on energy requirements.

How much fat is that? Check the following chart to see the amount of fat that equals 30 percent of calories.

Total kcal/d	Fat kcal/d	Grams of fat/d
1,200	360	40
1,500	450	50
1,600	480	53
1,800	540	60
2,000	600	67
2,500	750	83
3,000	900	100

How to calculate percent of fat

1. Check the nutrition label for grams of fat per serving.

2. Multiply the number of fat grams by 9 to get the number of calories from fat.

3. Divide the number of calories from fat by the number of calories in a serving.

4. Multiply this number by 100 to get the percent of calories from fat.

The goal is to consume about 30 percent of total calories from fat over the entire day. Some foods may be 50 percent fat, others 10 percent, as long as it balances to about 30 percent.

FIGURE 2.4   Determining daily fat intake.

Preliminary data suggests that there may be differences in protein requirements of male and female athletes. Protein intake is a concern of female athletes who are restricting calories to maintain low body weights or who are consuming vegetarian diets. Many female athletes also are overly concerned about fat. Although too much fat is not desirable, having a very low fat intake is also unhealthy. In an effort to reduce fat intake, athletes often omit entire food groups such as meat and dairy products. These food groups provide key nutrients for health and performance.

REFERENCES

1. Lagua, R. T., Claudio, V. S., and Thiele, V. F., *Nutrition and Diet Therapy Reference Dictionary*, Mosby, St. Louis, 1974, 162.
2. Williams, M. H., *Nutrition For Fitness and Sport*, 4th ed., Brown and Benchmark, Madison, 1995, 7.

3. Grandjean, A. C., Practices and recommendations of sports nutritionists, *Int. J. Sport Nutr.*, 3, 232, 1993.
4. Storlie, J., Nutrition assessment of athletes: A model for integrating nutrition and physical performance indicators, *Int. J. Sport Nutr.*, 1, 192, 1991.
5. U.S. Department of Agriculture and U.S. Department of Health and Human Services, The Dietary Guidelines for Americans, 2nd ed., U.S. Government Printing Office, Washington, D.C., 1989.
6. Hahn, N. I., Variety is still the spice of a healthful diet, *J. Am. Diet. Assoc.*, 95, 1096, 1995.
7. U.S. Department of Agriculture, The Food Pyramid, Washington, D.C., U.S. Government Printing Office, 1992.
8. Kennedy, E. T., Ohls, J., Carlson, S., and Fleming, K., The healthy eating index:design and applications, *J. Am. Diet. Assoc.*, 95, 1103, 1995.
9. Leaf, A. and Frisa, K. B., Eating for health or for athletic performance? *Am. J. Clin. Nutr.*, 49, 1066, 1989.
10. Jacobson, B. H. and Aldana, S. G., Current nutrition practice and knowledge of varsity athletes, *J. Appl. Sport Sci. Res.*, 6, 232, 1992.
11. Grandjean, A. C., unpublished data, 1991.
12. Bergstrom, J., Hermansen, L., Hultman, E., and Saltin, B., Diet, muscle glycogen and physical performance, *Acta. Physiol. Scand.* 71, 140, 1967.
13. Bergstrom, J. and Hultman, E., A study of the glycogen metabolism during exercise in man, *Scand. J. Clin. Invest.*, 19, 218, 1967.
14. Hermansen, L., Hultman, E., and Saltin, B., Muscle glycogen during prolonged severe exercise, *Acta. Physiol. Scand.*, 71, 129, 1967.
15. Sherman, W. M. and Wimer, G. S., Insufficient dietary carbohydrate during training: does it impair athletic performance? *Int. J. Sport Nutr.*, 1, 28, 1991.
16. Tanaka, J. A., Tanaka, H., and Landis, W., An assessment of carbohydrate intake in collegiate distance runners, *Int. J. Sport Nutr.*, 5, 206, 1995.
17. Economos, C. D., Bortz, S. S., and Nelson, M. E., Nutritional practices of elite athletes, *Sports Med.*, 16, 381, 1993.
18. Walberg-Rankin, J., Edmonds, C. E., and Gwazdauskas, F. C., Diet and weight changes of female bodybuilders before and after competition, *Int. J. Sport Nutr.*, 3, 87, 1993.
19. Nevill, M. E., Boobis, L. H., Brooks, S., and Williams, C., Effects of training on muscle metabolism during treadmill sprinting, *J. Appl. Physiol.*, 67, 2376, 1989.
20. Bangsbo, J., Norregaard, L., and Thorsoe, F., The effect of carbohydrate diet on intermittent exercise performance, *Int. J. Sports Med.*, 13, 152, 1992.
21. Hawley, J. A., Dennis, S. C., and Noakes, T. D., Carbohydrate, fluid, and electrolyte requirements of the soccer player: A review, *Int. J. Sport Nutr.*, 4, 221, 1994.
22. Jacobs, I., Westlin, N., Karlsson, J., Rasmusson, M., and Houghton, B., Muscle glycogen and diet in elite soccer players, *Eur. J. Appl. Physiol.*, 48, 297, 1982.
23. Sherman, W. M., Peden, M. C., Wright, D. A., Carbohydrate feeding 1 hr before exercise improves cycling performance, *Am. J. Clin. Nutr.*, 54, 866, 1991.
24. Sherman, W. M., Brodowicz, G., Wright, D. A., Allen, W. K., Simonsen, J., and Dernbach, A., Effects of 4 h preexercise carbohydrate feedings on cycling performance, *Med. Sci. Sports Exerc.*, 21, 598, 1989.
25. Jenkins, D. J. A., Wolever, T. M. S., Taylor, R. H., Barker, H., Fielden, H., Baldwin, J. M., Bowling, A. C., Newman, H. C., Jenkins, A. L., and Goff, D. V., Glycemic index of foods: a physiological basis for carbohydrate exchange, *Am. J. Clin. Nutr.*, 34, 362, 1981.
26. Horowitz, J. F., and Coyle, E. F., Metabolic responses to preexercise meals containing various carbohydrates and fat, *Am. J. Clin. Nutr.*, 58, 235, 1993.
27. Thomas, D. E., Brotherhood, J. R., and Brand, J. C., Carbohydrate feedings before exercise: effect of glycemic index, *Int. J. Sports Med.*, 12, 180, 1991.
28. Coyle, E. F., Coggan, A. R., Hemmert, M. K., and Ivy, J. L., Muscle glycogen utilization during prolonged strenuous exercise when fed carbohydrate, *J. Appl. Physiol.*, 61, 165, 1986.

29. Coyle, E. F., Hagberg, J. M., Hurley, B. F., Martin, W. H., Ehsani, A. A., and Holloszy, J. O., Carbohydrate feedings during prolonged strenuous exercise can delay fatigue, *J. Appl. Physiol.*, 55, 230, 1983.

30. Wright, D. A., Sherman, W. M., Dernbach, A. R., Carbohydrate feedings before, during, or in combination improve cycling endurance performance, *J. Appl. Physiol.*, 71, 1082, 1991.

31. Costill, D. L. and Hargreaves, M., Carbohydrate nutrition and fatigue, *Sports Med.*, 13, 86, 1992.

32. Coggan, A. R. and Coyle, E. F., Effect of carbohydrate feedings during high-intensity exercise, *J. Appl. Physiol.*, 65, 1703, 1988.

33. Lugo, M., Sherman, W. M., Wimer, G. S., and Garleb, K., Metabolic responses when different forms of carbohydrate energy are consumed during cycling, *Int. J. Sport Nutr.*, 3, 398, 1993.

34. Coyle, E. F., Substrate utilization during exercise in active people, *Am. J. Clin. Nutr.*, 61, 968S, 1995.

35. Coleman, E., Update on carbohydrate: solid vs. liquid, *Int. J. Sport Nutr.*, 4, 80, 1994.

36. Ivy, J. L., Katz, A. L., Cutler, C. L., Sherman, W. M. and Coyle, E. F., Muscle glycogen synthesis after exercise: effect of time of carbohydrate ingestion, *J. Appl Physiol.*, 64, 1480, 1988.

37. Ivy, J. L., Lee, M. C., Brozinick, J. T., and Reed, M. J., Muscle glycogen storage after different amounts of carbohydrate ingestion, *J. Appl. Physiol.*, 65, 2018, 1988.

38. Reed, M. J., Brozinick, J. T., Lee, M. C., and Ivy, J. L., Muscle glycogen storage postexercise: effect of mode of carbohydrate administration, *J. Appl. Physiol.*, 66, 720, 1989.

39. Blom, P. C. S., Hostmark, A. T., Vaage, O., Kardel, K. R., and Maehlum, S., Effect of different post-exercise sugar diets on the rate of muscle glycogen synthesis, *Med. Sci. Sports Exerc.*, 19, 491, 1987.

40. Burke, L. M., Collier, G. R., and Hargreaves, M., Muscle glycogen storage after prolonged exercise: effect of the glycemic index of carbohydrate feedings, *J. Appl. Physiol.*, 75, 1019, 1993.

41. Sherman, W. M., Costill, D. L., Fink, W. J., and Miller, J. M., Effect of exercise-diet manipulation on muscle glycogen and its subsequent use during performance, *Int. J. Sports Med.*, 2, 114, 1981.

42. Burke, L. M. and Read, R. S. D., A study of carbohydrate loading techniques used by marathon runners, *Can. J. Sport Sci.*, 12, 6, 1987.

43. Tarnopolsky, M. A., Atkinson, S. A., Phillips, S. M., and MacDougall, J. D., Carbohydrate loading and metabolism during exercise in men and women, *J. Appl. Physiol.*, 78, 1360, 1995.

44. Young, V. R. and Pellett, P. L., Plant proteins in relation to human protein and amino acid nutrition, *Am. J. Clin. Nutr.*, 59, 1203S, 1994.

45. Position of the American Dietetic Association: Vegetarian Diets, *J. Am. Diet. Assoc.*, 93, 1317, 1993.

46. Lemon, P. W. R., Do athletes need more dietary protein and amino acids? *Int. J. Sport Nutr.*, 5, S39, 1995.

47. Lemon, P. W. R., Influence of dietary protein and total energy intake on strength improvement, *Sports Science Exchange*, Gatorade Sports Science Institute, 2, April, 1989.

48. Lemon, P. W. R. and Nagle, F. J., Effects of exercise on protein and amino acid metabolism, *Med. Sci. Sports Exerc.*, 13, 141, 1981.

49. Millward, D. J., Davies, C. T. M., Halliday, D., Wolman, S. L., Matthews, D., and Rennie, M., Effect of exercise on protein metabolism in humans as explored with stable isotopes, *Fed. Proc.*, 41, 2686, 1982.

50. Lemon, P. W. R. and Mullin, J. P., Effect of initial muscle glycogen levels on protein catabolism during exercise, *J. Appl. Physiol.*, 48, 624, 1980.

51. Butterfield, G. E., Whole-body protein utilization in humans, *Med. Sci. Sports Exerc.*, 19, S157, 1987.

52. Butterfield, G. E., and Calloway, D. H., Physical activity improves protein utilization, *Br. J. Nutr.*, 51, 171, 1984.
53. Friedman, J. E. and Lemon, P. W. R., Effect of chronic endurance exercise on retention of dietary protein, *Int. J. Sports Med.*, 10, 118, 1989.
54. Meredith, C. N., Zackin, M. J., Frontera, W. R., and Evans, W. J., Dietary protein requirements and body protein metabolism in endurance-trained men, *J. Appl. Physiol.*, 66, 2850, 1989.
55. Tarnopolsky, M. A., MacDougall, J. D., and Atkinson, S. A., Influence of protein intake and training status on nitrogen balance and lean body mass, *J. Appl. Physiol.*, 64, 187, 1988.
56. Brouns, F., Saris, W. H. M., Stroecken, J., Beckers, E., Thijssen, R., Rehrer, N. J., and ten Hoor, F., The effect of diet manipulation and repeated sustained exercise on nitrogen balance, a controlled Tour de France simulation study, Part 3, In Brouns, F., (Ed.), *Food and Fluid Related Aspects in Highly Trained Athletes*, Haarlem, The Netherlands: De Vrieseborch, 1988, 73.
57. Tarnopolsky, L. J., Tarnopolsky, M. A., Atkinson, S. A., and MacDougall, J. D., Gender differences in metabolic responses to endurance exercise, *J. Appl. Physiol.*, 68, 302, 1990.
58. Phillips, S. M., Atkinson, S. A., Tarnopolsky, M. A., and MacDougall, J. D., *J. Appl. Physiol.*, 75, 2134, 1993.
59. Harris, H. A., Nutrition and Physical Performance, *Proc. of the Nutr. Soc.*, 25, 87, 1966.
60. McArdle, W. D., Katch, F. J., and Katch, V. L., *Exercise Physiology: Energy, Nutrition, and Human Performance*, Lea and Febiger, Philadelphia, 1986, 290.
61. Gontzea, I., Sutzescu, R., and Dumitrache, S., The influence of adaptation to physical effort on nitrogen balance in man, *Nutr. Rep. Int.*, 11, 231, 1975.
62. Cohen, J. L., Potosnak, L., Frank, O., and Baker, H., A nutritional and hematological assessment of elite ballet dancers, *Phys. Sportsmed.*, 13, 43, 1985.
63. Keith, R. E., O'Keeffe, K. A., Lynn, A. A., and Young, K. L., Dietary status of trained female cyclists, *J. Am. Diet. Assoc.*, 89, 1620, 1989.
64. Kaiserauer, S., Snyder, A. C., Sleeper, M., and Zierath, J., Nutritional, physiological, and menstrual status of distance runners, *Med. Sci. Sports Exerc.*, 21, 120, 1989.
65. Lamar-Hildebrand, N., Saldanha, L., and Endres, J., Dietary and exercise practices of college-aged female bodybuilders, *J. Am. Diet. Assoc.*, 89, 1308, 1989.
66. Barr, S. I., Nutrition knowledge and selected nutritional practices of female recreational athletes, *J. Nutr. Edu.*, 18, 167, 1986.
67. Slavin, J. L. and McNamara, E. A., Nutritional practices of women cyclists, including recreational riders and elite racers, In *Sport, Health and Nutrition*, Vol 2, Broekhoff, J., Ellis, M. J., and Tripps D. G. (Eds.), Human Kinetics, Champaign, 1986.
68. Krizmanic, J., Here's who we are, *Vegetarian Times*, October, 72, 1992.
69. Dwyer, J. T., Vegetarian eating patterns: science, values, and food choices — where do we go from here? *Am. J. Clin. Nutr.*, 59, 1255S, 1994.
70. Young, V. R., Soy protein in relation to human protein and amino acid nutrition, *J. Am. Diet. Assoc.*, 91, 828, 1991.
71. Carlson, E., Kipps, M., Lockie, A., and Thompson, J., A comparative evaluation of vegan, vegetarian and omnivore diets, *J. Plant Foods*, 6, 89, 1985.
72. Janelle, K. C. and Barr, S. I., Nutrient intakes and eating behavior scores of vegetarian and nonvegetarian women, *J. Am. Diet Assoc.*, 95, 180, 1995.
73. Grundy, S. M., Monounsaturated fatty acids and cholesterol metabolism: implications for dietary recommendations, *J. Nutr.*, 119, 529, 1989.
74. Summary of the second report of the National Cholesterol Education Program (NCEP), Expert panel on detection, evaluation and treatment of high blood cholesterol in adults (Adult Treatment Panel II), *J. Am. Med. Assoc.*, 269, 3015, 1993.
75. Costill, D. L., Coyle, E. F., Dalsky, G., Evans, W., Fink, W., and Hoopes, D., Effects of elevated plasma FFA and insulin on muscle glycogen usage during exercise, *J. Appl. Physiol.*, 43, 695, 1977.

76. Vukovich, M. D., Costill, D. L., Hickey, M. S., Trappe, S. W., Cole, K. J., and Fink, W. J., Effect of fat emulsion infusion and fat feeding on muscle glycogen utilization during cycle exercise, *J. Appl. Physiol.*, 75, 1513, 1993.

77. Essen, B., Intramuscular substrate utilization during prolonged exercise, *Ann. N.Y. Acad. Sci.*, 301, 30, 1977.

78. Askew, E. W., Fat metabolism in exercise, In *Nutrient Utilization During Exercise*, Ross Symposium on Nutrient Utilization During Exercise, Ross Laboratories, Columbus, 1984, 13.

79. Jansson, E. and Kaijser, L., Substrate utilization and enzymes in skeletal muscle of extremely endurance-trained men, *J. Appl. Physiol.*, 62, 999, 1987.

80. Ruby, B. C., and Robergs, R. A., Gender differences in substrate utilization during exercise, *Sports Med.*, 17, 393, 1994.

81. *Healthy People 2000:National Health Promotion and Disease Prevention Objectives,* Washington, D.C., U.S. Department of Health and Human Services, 1990.

82. Lewis, C. J., Crane, N. T., Moore, B. J., and Hubbard, V. S., Healthy people 2000:Report on the 1994 nutrition progress review, *Nutrition Today*, 29, 6, 1994.

83. Kris-Etherton, P. M. and Krummel, D., Role of nutrition in the prevention and treatment of coronary heart disease in women, *J. Am. Diet. Assoc.*, 93, 987, 1993.

84. Hankin, J. H., Role of nutrition in women's health: Diet and breast cancer, *J. Am. Diet. Assoc.*, 93, 994, 1993.

85. St Jeor, S. T., The role of weight management in the health of women, *J. Am. Diet. Assoc.*, 93, 1007, 1993.

86. McDowell, M. A., Briefel, R. R., Alaimo, K., Bischof, A. M., Caughman, C. R., Carroll, M. D., Loria, C. M., and Johnson, C. L., Energy and macronutrient intakes of persons ages 2 months and over in the United States: Third National Health and Nutrition Examination Survey, Phase 1, 1988-1991, Advance data from vital and health statistics; No 255, Hyattsville, Maryland: National Center for Health Statistics, 1994.

87. Nestel, P. J., Contribution of fats and fatty acids to performance of the elite athlete, in *Nutrition and Fitness for Athletes*, Simopoulos, A. P. and Pavlou, K. N., (Eds.) World Rev. Nutr. Diet., Basel, Karger, 1993, 61.

88. Sherman, W. M. and Leenders, N., Fat loading: The next magic bullet? *Int. J. Sport Nutr.*, 5, S1, 1995.

THE VITAMINS

CONTENTS

I. INTRODUCTION

Vitamins regulate many processes in the body. They are generally divided into two classes: fat-soluble and water-soluble. The fat-soluble vitamins are A, D, E, and K; the water-soluble vitamins include the B-complex vitamins and vitamin C. Although each vitamin has unique functions, a few characteristics generally distinguish the two groups (Table 3.1).

Water-soluble vitamins act as coenzymes in energy production and metabolism of carbohydrates, protein, and fat. Because they are not stored to any

TABLE 3.1   The Vitamins

Nutrient	Functions	Sources	RDA[a]
Water-Soluble			
Thiamin	Part of a coenzyme used in energy metabolism; maintains nervous system and appetite	Whole grains, pork, legumes, seeds, and nuts	1.1 mg
Riboflavin	Part of a coenzyme used in energy metabolism; supports normal vision, and healthy skin	Dairy products, leafy green vegetables, enriched breads and cereals	1.3 mg
Niacin	Part of a coenzyme used in energy metabolism; supports healthy skin, nervous system, and gastrointestinal tract	Protein foods such as meat, milk, eggs, fish, and poultry	15 mg NE
Vitamin B_6	Part of a coenzyme used in amino acid and fatty acid metabolism. Helps convert tryptophan to niacin. Helps make red blood cells	Meat, fish, poultry, green leafy vegetables, fruits, whole grains	1.6 mg
Folate	DNA and RNA synthesis; amino acid metabolism	Green leafy vegetables, legumes, nuts, beef liver	180 µg[b]
Vitamin B_{12}	DNA synthesis; used in blood formation, helps maintain nerve tissue	Animal products (meat, fish, poultry, eggs, milk, cheese)	2.0 mg
Vitamin C	Antioxidant, collagen synthesis; strengthens resistance to infection, helps in absorption of iron	Citrus fruits, vegetables such as broccoli, cabbage, and potatoes; cantaloupe, strawberries, and tomatoes	60 mg
Fat-Soluble			
Vitamin A	Important for proper vision, reproduction, healthy skin, and regulation of hormones	Fortified milk, butter, eggs, liver, margarine	800 µg RE
Beta-carotene	Antioxidant, precursor of vitamin A; plays an important role in disease prevention	Green leafy vegetables such as broccoli and spinach; apricots, cantaloupe, squash, carrots, sweet potatoes, pumpkin	30 mg[c]
Vitamin E	Antioxidant, regulator of oxidative reactions	Vegetable oils, wheat germ, nuts, legumes, green leafy vegetables	8 mg α-TE
Vitamin D	Promotes normal bone and teeth formation; regulates the absorption of calcium	Fortified milk, margarine, eggs, liver, sardines	10 µg
Vitamin K	Blood clotting, a blood protein that regulates blood calcium	Liver, green leafy vegetables; synthesized in the gut	65 µg

[a]   Except where indicated all RDAs reflect amounts established for 19–24 year-old females.
[b]   Some health experts recommend up to 400 µg/d to help prevent neural tube defects in the developing fetus during pregnancy.
[c]   Beneficial amount.

degree in the body, they are required daily in small amounts in the diet. Once the body has all it needs, excess amounts of water-soluble vitamins are excreted in the urine.[1] This is why many athletes believe that water-soluble vitamins are safe to consume in large amounts. However, some water-soluble vitamins such as vitamin B_6 and niacin are reportedly toxic at high doses.[2,3] Because the B-complex vitamins and vitamin C are soluble in water, they are easily destroyed during preparation, cooking, or storage.

Fat-soluble vitamins do not function as coenzymes but have different mechanisms of action. They are soluble in fat and are stored in the liver and other fatty tissues in the body. The fat-soluble vitamins perform many important functions. For example, vitamin A is essential for night vision. Vitamin D promotes the absorption of calcium and phosphorus and thus is important to bone health. Vitamin E is an antioxidant that prevents cell membrane damage. Vitamin K aids in blood clotting.

Because the fat-soluble vitamins are not closely involved in energy metabolism or muscle growth, the addition of these vitamins to an already adequate diet is not likely to affect performance.[4] However, data suggests that vitamin E, as an antioxidant, may reduce oxidative damage to red blood cells and muscle tissue during high intensity exercise.[5]

True vitamin deficiency diseases are rare today because many foods are enriched and fortified with vitamins. However, it becomes increasingly difficult to meet daily requirements for all vitamins if an athlete does not consume enough calories to meet energy needs or has a diet consistently lacking in several nutrients. Dietary surveys of female athletes have reported low dietary intakes of several vitamins including the fat-soluble vitamins D and E, and the water-soluble vitamins thiamin, niacin, riboflavin, vitamin B_6, folic acid, and vitamin B_{12}. Therefore, the following discussion will include these vitamins which are of particular importance to female athletes.

II. FAT-SOLUBLE VITAMINS

A. VITAMIN D

Vitamin D (calciferol) belongs to a class of substances known as sterols. All sterols, such as cholesterol, are made by the body, except for vitamin D. Ultraviolet light from the sun is needed to convert an inactive substance found in the skin and in food into active vitamin D.

The major function of vitamin D is to enhance the absorption of calcium and phosphorus. Vitamin D is also necessary for reproduction and growth.[6] As research advances, it is likely that vitamin D may play an important role in the treatment of various diseases including osteoporosis, breast cancer, and psoriasis.[7]

A deficiency of vitamin D results in poor absorption of calcium and phosphorus. Without adequate vitamin D, bones demineralize and become porous and weak. In children, this condition is known as rickets, a disease characterized by abnormal bone growth that can result in bowed legs and other deformities.[8]

Adult rickets, or osteomalacia, occurs most frequently in women who have low calcium intakes and little exposure to sunlight. For most people, particularly the elderly, sunlight is the most important contributor to vitamin D requirements.[7] Ultraviolet light catalyzes the synthesis of vitamin D_3 (cholecalciferol) from 7-dehydrocholesterol, which can then be used by the body.[9] Many factors, including seasonal changes, time of day, sunscreen use, and skin pigmentation can influence the production of vitamin D in the skin.[9] For example, in the summertime in the U.S., our skin synthesizes six International Units (IU) vitamin $D/cm^2/h$. The rate decreases to one fourth of that in the wintertime.[9]

Vitamin D is not found in great supply in foods. Some is present in small amounts in liver, butter, and egg yolk. Milk which is fortified with 400 IU of vitamin D per quart contributes most of the vitamin D in our food supply. The RDA for vitamin D is 10 μg/d cholecalciferol (400 IU) for females up to age 25, after which the RDA decreases to 5 μg/d (200 IU) of cholecalciferol.[10]

Low vitamin D intakes have been reported among some groups of female athletes. Lamar-Hildebrand et al.[11] studied the dietary practices of female bodybuilders and reported a mean vitamin D intake of less than 66% of the RDA. To achieve low body-fat levels, bodybuilders often exclude foods they believe contain a lot of fat such as egg yolk, butter, and milk, foods that supply vitamin D. In another study involving elite ballet dancers, Cohen et al.[12] reported a low mean vitamin D intake (less than 25% of the RDA). The female dancers avoided dairy products in order to cut calories, which most likely contributed to their inadequate intake.

It is important that female athletes understand that milk and other dairy products are not especially high in calories and/or fat if consumed in moderation. Milk is a good source of vitamin D and calcium along with other essential nutrients. Inadequate dietary calcium and vitamin D can result in weak bones and increased risk for osteoporosis.[13] Even more immediate is the risk of stress fractures which can force an athlete out of competition.

Compared with other fat-soluble vitamins, vitamin D is considered highly toxic. Excess intakes of vitamin D can produce high blood calcium levels and calcium deposits in soft tissue, resulting in irreversible kidney and cardiovascular damage.[14] Symptoms of vitamin D toxicity include thirst, polyuria, muscle weakness, joint pain, nausea, and vomiting.[15]

B. VITAMIN E

Vitamin E is known chemically as an antioxidant. It protects the body from free radicals, substances that can damage cells and tissues. Free radicals are produced by the body's own metabolism and can be generated from exposure to environmental factors such as pollution, cigarette smoke, radiation, and some drugs and pesticides. When free radicals attack cell membranes, they promote a harmful process known as lipid peroxidation. Vitamin E serves as one of the body's first defenders against lipid perioxidation by breaking the free radical chain reaction.[16]

The RDA for vitamin E is 8 mg/d alpha-tocopherol α-TE for women. The need for vitamin E depends on the type of dietary fat consumed and the presence or absence of other antioxidants.[17] Polyunsaturated fatty acids increase the requirement for vitamin E while antioxidants such as selenium and vitamin C decrease the requirement for vitamin E.[18]

The richest sources of vitamin E are found primarily in polyunsaturated vegetable oils such as soybean, corn, cottonseed, and safflower. Other good sources include dark green leafy vegetables, wheat germ, nuts, and legumes.

Compared to other fat-soluble vitamins, vitamin E is relatively nontoxic. Few sides effects have been reported, even at amounts as high as 3200 IU/d, which is about 400 times the RDA.[19] With the recent popularity of vitamin E and its effect as an antioxidant, increased consumption of this vitamin is likely and therefore further research is needed on its safety at high doses.

1. The Role of Vitamin E in Exercise

Studies have shown that strenuous exercise may promote free radical production, leading to lipid peroxidation and tissue damage.[20] During strenuous exercise, oxygen consumption in the exercising muscle can increase as much as 10- to 40-fold over the resting state.[20] This increased use of oxygen can produce minor muscle tissue damage. Vitamin E may protect against such damage or at least help reduce it by interrupting the chain reaction of lipid peroxidation, which can destroy cell membranes.[21]

One study[5] examined the effect of antioxidants on muscle damage in trained and untrained individuals. Ten healthy subjects took a supplement containing vitamin E, vitamin C, and beta-carotene for 6 weeks and were compared to ten subjects who did not take the supplement. Those who took the antioxidant supplement showed less free radical production at rest and after exercise, which may have averted muscle damage. In another study,[22] elite endurance athletes who took antioxidant vitamins for four weeks had less muscle damage after exercise than a control group.

Although research is encouraging, the functions that free radicals and vitamin E perform in the body remain unclear. Free radicals are certainly not the cause of exercise-induced muscle damage, and taking antioxidants such as vitamin E is not the solution. A certain amount of free radical production is necessary for normal tissue growth. Additionally, while vitamin E may protect the muscles from daily wear and tear, there is little data showing that supplementation with vitamin E improves performance, except perhaps in athletes exercising at high altitudes.[23]

Simon-Schnass and Pabst[23] investigated the effects of vitamin E supplementation on physical performance and cell damage in 12 mountain climbers. Subjects were randomly assigned to either a supplement group receiving

400 mg/d of vitamin E for 4 weeks or a placebo group. The amount of exhaled pentane was measured before and after supplementation. Pentane is one of the hydrocarbon gases produced during lipid peroxidation. After 4 weeks of vitamin E supplementation, exhaled pentane increased more than 100% in the placebo group, but decreased in the treatment group. It was concluded that vitamin E supplementation had a beneficial effect on physical performance and tissue protection at high altitudes.

Because strenuous exercise may promote free radical formation, it has been suggested that endurance athletes may benefit from more vitamin E. Simon-Schnass[25] approves of 100 to 200 IU/d of vitamin E for athletes who begin a more strenuous training program, especially at high altitudes. However, more studies are needed to determine the effects of vitamin E on physical performance.

III. WATER-SOLUBLE VITAMINS

A. THIAMIN

Thiamin, a component of the coenzyme thiamin pyrophosphate (TPP), is essential for the metabolism of carbohydrates and certain amino acids. Thiamin also plays a role in cell reproduction and normal functioning of the nervous system.

The need for thiamin is related to energy intake. Thiamin requirements increase in relative proportion to higher energy intakes. Sauberlich et al.[26] studied thiamin requirements of subjects consuming either 2800 kcal/d or 3600 kcal/d and reported that at the higher caloric level, a minimum of 0.3 mg of thiamin per 1000 kcal/d was necessary to maintain normal thiamin levels.

There is also a direct relationship between carbohydrate intake and thiamin requirements.[26] As the carbohydrate content of the diet increases, so does the need for thiamin. Thus, athletes consuming high-calorie, high-carbohydrate diets may have increased thiamin requirements.[27]

The RDA for thiamin is 0.5 mg/1000 kcal/d and no less than 1.0 mg/d for those consuming 2000 calories or less.[28] Females need approximately 1.1 mg/d of thiamin. Whole grain foods including breads, cereals, pasta, and rice supply almost half the thiamin in women's diets. Good sources of thiamin include lean pork, liver, fish, poultry, egg yolk, cheese, legumes, wheat germ, and green, leafy vegetables. Most ready-to-eat and instant-prepared cereals are fortified with thiamin. Table 3.2 shows food sources of thiamin.

B. RIBOFLAVIN

Riboflavin functions as part of two coenzymes, flavin mononucleotide and flavin adenine dinucleotide, that are involved in energy metabolism. Riboflavin is important for normal vision and for maintaining healthy skin.

TABLE 3.2

Food Sources of Thiamin ✍

RDA for women: 1.1 mg/d

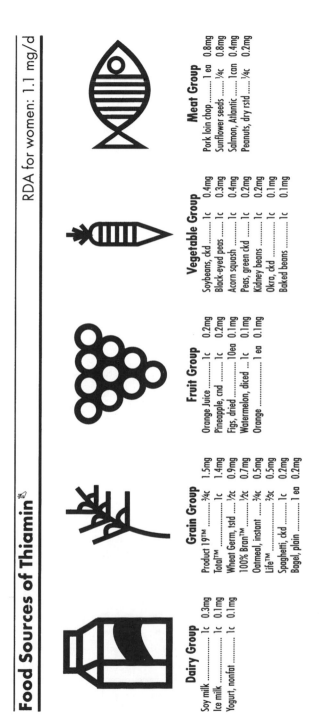

Dairy Group

Soy milk	1c	0.3mg
Ice milk	1c	0.1mg
Yogurt, nonfat	1c	0.1mg

Grain Group

Product 19™	¾c	1.5mg
Total™	1c	1.4mg
Wheat Germ, tstd	½c	0.9mg
100% Bran™	½c	0.7mg
Oatmeal, instant	¾c	0.5mg
Life™	⅔c	0.5mg
Spaghetti, ckd	1c	0.2mg
Bagel, plain	1 ea	0.2mg

Fruit Group

Orange Juice	1c	0.2mg
Pineapple, cnd	1c	0.2mg
Figs, dried	10ea	0.1mg
Watermelon, diced	1c	0.1mg
Orange	1 ea	0.1mg

Vegetable Group

Soybeans, ckd	1c	0.4mg
Black-eyed peas	1c	0.3mg
Acorn squash	1c	0.4mg
Peas, green ckd	1c	0.2mg
Kidney beans	1c	0.2mg
Okra, ckd	1c	0.1mg
Baked beans	1c	0.1mg

Meat Group

Pork loin chop	1 ea	0.8mg
Sunflower seeds	¼c	0.8mg
Salmon, Atlantic	1 can	0.4mg
Peanuts, dry rstd	¼c	0.2mg

✍*An excellent source provides more than 0.2 mg per serving*

The RDA for riboflavin is 1.3 mg/d for females or approximately 0.6 mg/1000 kcal/d.[29] During pregnancy and lactation, riboflavin requirements increase to 1.6 mg/d and 1.8 mg/d, respectively.

In the U.S., approximately one fourth of the riboflavin in women's diets comes from milk and dairy products, meat, fish, and poultry. Cereals and flours are generally low in riboflavin, unless they are enriched or fortified. Although fruits and vegetables are fair sources of this vitamin, they are not consumed in adequate amounts to satisfy daily requirements. Table 3.3 shows food sources of riboflavin.

Female athletes who have low energy intakes and limit their intake of red meat may have difficulty meeting riboflavin requirements. In a study of female distance runners, Kaiserauer et al.[30] reported that riboflavin intakes were significantly lower in amenorrheic female runners than in regularly menstruating subjects. Compared to regularly menstruating athletes, amenorrheic athletes consumed fewer calores, 2490 kcal/d and 1582 kcal/d, respectively. None of the amenorrheic athletes consumed red meat.

Previous studies have indicated that active women may require more riboflavin than the RDA.[31,32] However, female athletes can obtain adequate amounts of riboflavin through the diet.[33] Riboflavin supplementation is not necessary and most likely will not improve performance.[34]

C. NIACIN

The vitamin niacin, like thiamin and riboflavin, plays an important role in energy metabolism. It is made up of two coenzymes, nicotinamide adenine dinucleotide (NAD) and nicotinamide adenine dinucleotide phosphate (NADP).

Niacin can be formed in the body from tryptophan, an essential amino acid found in meat, poultry, fish, and eggs. A diet providing the RDA for protein should supply enough niacin even if the diet itself is low in niacin. The RDA is 15 mg NE (niacin equivalents) a day for women 11 to 50 years of age.[35] One niacin equivalent is equal to 60 mg of tryptophan.

Good sources of niacin include enriched cereals and pasta, chicken, tuna, and peanut butter (Table 3.4). Although milk and eggs contain only small amounts of niacin, they are rich sources of tryptophan and thus contribute to total daily niacin intake.

It is unlikely that athletes consuming a variety of foods will develop a niacin deficiency. Diets providing low levels of niacin equivalents and other B-complex vitamins over time, however, can produce a deficiency state. Early signs include fatigue, listlessness, headache, backache, and loss of appetite.

Niacin is widely available as an over-the-counter supplement, and is one of the least expensive drugs used for treating high blood cholesterol levels. In daily doses of 2 to 3 g, nicotinic acid reportedly reduces total cholesterol and low-density lipoprotein cholesterol levels by 20 to 30%.[36] However, research

TABLE 3.3

Food Sources of Riboflavin 🐑

RDA for women: 1.3 mg/d

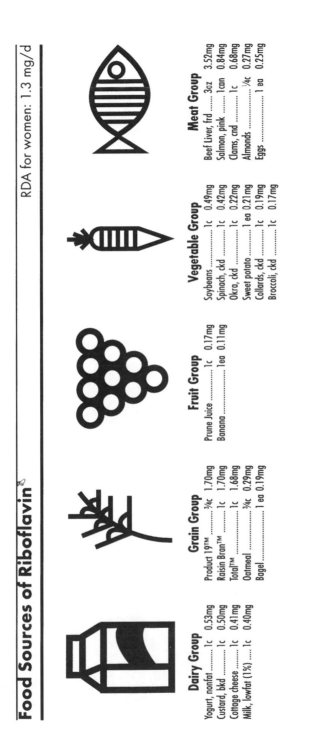

Dairy Group
Yogurt, nonfat	1c	0.53mg
Custard, bkd	1c	0.50mg
Cottage cheese	1c	0.41mg
Milk, lowfat (1%)	1c	0.40mg

Grain Group
Product 19™	¾c	1.70mg
Raisin Bran™	1c	1.70mg
Total™	1c	1.68mg
Oatmeal	¾c	0.29mg
Bagel	1 ea	0.19mg

Fruit Group
Prune Juice	1c	0.17mg
Banana	1 ea	0.11mg

Vegetable Group
Soybeans	1c	0.49mg
Spinach, ckd	1c	0.42mg
Okra, ckd	1c	0.22mg
Sweet potato	1 ea	0.21mg
Collards, ckd	1c	0.19mg
Broccoli, ckd	1c	0.17mg

Meat Group
Beef Liver, frd	3oz	3.52mg
Salmon, pink	1 can	0.84mg
Clams, cnd	1c	0.68mg
Almonds	¼c	0.27mg
Eggs	1 ea	0.25mg

🐑 *An excellent source provides more than 0.2 mg per serving*

TABLE 3.4

Food Sources of Niacin    RDA for women: 15 mg NE/d

Dairy Group

Instant bkfast, dry .	1 env	5.00mg
Soy milk	1 c	0.35mg
Blue cheese	1 oz	0.28mg
Milk, skim	1 c	0.21mg

Grain Group

Product 19™	¾ c	20.00mg
Total™	1 c	19.80mg
Oatmeal, instant	¾ c	5.90mg

Fruit Group

Prunes, dried	10ea	1.65mg
Peaches, frozen	1 c	1.63mg
Avocado, Florida	¼ c	1.46mg
Apricots, dr	10ea	1.05mg
Strawberries, frzn .	1 c	1.02mg
Orange Juice	1 c	0.99mg
Fruit cocktail, cnd ..	1 c	1.00mg

Vegetable Group

Mushrooms, ckd	½ c	3.4mg
Potato, bkd	1 ea	3.3mg
Green peas, ckd	1 c	3.2mg
Potatoes, mashed	1 c	2.3mg
Baked beans, ckd	1 c	0.8mg

Meat Group

Salmon, w/bones ..	1 can	29.7mg
Tuna, water/pkd	1 can	26.0mg
Chicken breast	1 ea	12.5mg
Beef liver, fried	3 oz	12.3mg
Swordfish, bkd	3 oz	10.0mg
Peanuts, roasted	¼ c	5.1mg
Peanut butter	2T	4.2mg

🐟 *An excellent source provides more than 3.0 mg per serving* has shown adverse reactions to large doses of niacin, which raises concern about the safety of niacin supplementation for health or performance reasons.[3]

D. VITAMIN B$_6$

Vitamin B$_6$ is made up of three chemically related compounds: pyridoxine, pyridoxal, and pyridoxamine. All three forms of vitamin B$_6$ are readily absorbed and converted to pyridoxal phosphate, the coenzyme necessary for metabolizing proteins and amino acids.

One of the most important functions of vitamin B$_6$ is its role in forming niacin from the amino acid tryptophan. The coenzyme pyridoxal phosphate helps transfer amino groups from one compound to another. Vitamin B$_6$ is also important for the synthesis of hemoglobin, the oxygen-carrying part of red blood cells, and for proper functioning of the nervous system.

Several dietary factors influence vitamin B$_6$ requirements, including bio-availability, caloric intake, carbohydrate intake, and protein intake.[37] The requirement for vitamin B$_6$ is directly related to protein. As protein intake increases, so does the need for vitamin B$_6$. The RDA for vitamin B$_6$ is based on the ratio of 0.016 mg vitamin B$_6$/g of dietary protein or 1.6 mg/d for females. This amount is adequate for women who consume an average of 60 g/d of protein.[38]

Foods from animal and plant sources provide about 48% and 52% of the total vitamin B$_6$ intake in the U.S. population, respectively.[39] Chicken, tuna, bananas, and avocados provide more than 0.4 mg per 3 oz. serving (Table 3.5). Although beef and milk supply small amounts of vitamin B$_6$, they are consumed often enough that they become important sources of vitamin B$_6$.

A deficiency of vitamin B$_6$ is most often seen in individuals who are also deficient in other B-complex vitamins.[40] Early deficiency symptoms include depression, dizziness, nausea, weight loss, and irritability.

Studies examining the nutrient intakes of female athletes have reported low dietary intakes of vitamin B$_6$ in runners,[41] cyclists,[42] gymnasts,[43] basketball players,[44] ice skaters,[45] and dancers.[12] Many of these studies, however, were conducted before 1989 and compared nutrient data with the 1980 RDAs. As previously mentioned in 1989, allowances for vitamin B$_6$ for women were reduced from 2.0 to 1.6 mg/d. Nevertheless, inadequate vitamin B$_6$ intakes are still being reported. Bergen-Cico and Short[46] published a study on adolescent female cross-country runners comparing nutrient data with the 1989 RDAs. The mean nutrient intake of vitamin B$_6$ was 1 mg/d, representing 65% of the RDA.

Few studies have conducted biochemical analyses or laboratory tests on blood or urine samples of athletes to determine vitamin B$_6$ status. Biochemical analyses reveal important facts about how the body uses specific nutrients. Low blood vitamin B$_6$ levels can indicate that dietary intake of vitamin B$_6$ is low or poorly absorbed, or that an individual has a higher requirement for vitamin B$_6$.

TABLE 3.5

Food Sources of Vitamin B₆ ✐

RDA for women: 1.6 mg/d

Dairy Group

Cottage cheese	1c	0.17mg
Ice milk	1c	0.13mg
Yogurt, nonfat	1c	0.12mg

Grain Group

Oatmeal, instant	¾c	0.74mg
Brown rice, ckd	1c	0.28mg

Fruit Group

Banana	1 ea	0.65mg
Prune Juice	½c	0.27mg
Pineapple Juice	1c	0.24mg
Watermelon	1c	0.23mg

Vegetable Group

Garbanzo beans	1c	1.14mg
Avocado, Florida	½ ea	0.80mg
Potato, bkd	1 ea	0.70mg
Prune juice	1c	0.55mg
Acorn squash	1c	0.47mg
Spinach, ckd	1c	0.43mg
Soybeans, ckd	1c	0.40mg
Lentils, ckd	1c	0.35mg
Baked beans	1c	0.34mg

Meat Group

Salmon, ckd	3oz	1.50mg
Beef liver, frd	3oz	1.22mg
Tuna, water/pkd	1 can	0.62mg
Chicken breast	3oz	0.51mg
Turkey, rstd	3oz	0.45mg
Sunflower seeds	¼c	0.40mg
Pork chop	1 ea.	0.34mg

✐ An excellent source provides more than 0.3 mg per serving

Rokitzki et al.[47] determined the vitamin B_6 status of strength and power athletes (12 women, 45 men) by means of a 7-day weighed food intake record and determination of vitamin B_6 in the blood. Results showed that athletes did not achieve the recommended amount of vitamin B_6 in the diet. Additionally, blood concentrations were below the normal range for vitamin B_6.

1. The Role of Vitamin B_6 In Exercise

Because vitamin B_6 plays a role in energy production, it has been suggested that the requirement for this vitamin is increased in active people.[48] This theory is based on evidence showing that exercise produces a significant increase in plasma concentrations of pyridoxal phosphate. Manore et al.[49] found this to be true regardless of the level of carbohydrate or vitamin B_6 in the diet. Crozier et al.[50] also reported a 14% increase in plasma pyridoxal phosphate in subjects maintaining adequate vitamin B_6 status.

Despite increases in vitamin B_6 during exercise, there are no well-documented studies showing that exercise increases the loss of vitamin B_6 from the body at a rate greater than can be easily replaced by eating foods that are good sources of vitamin B_6.[48] Furthermore, there is little data demonstrating that vitamin B_6 supplementation will improve performance in athletes consuming a well balanced diet.

2. Premenstrual Syndrome and Vitamin B_6

Vitamin B_6 has been a popular nutritional supplement used to relieve symptoms of premenstrual syndrome (PMS). Arguments for treating PMS with vitamin B_6 are based on its role as a coenzyme and its association with low levels of the neurotransmitter serotonin and depression.[51] According to some, increasing vitamin B_6 intake may elevate serotonin levels and thus decrease psychological and physical symptoms associated with PMS.[52]

Williams et al.[53] found significant improvements in PMS symptoms in women receiving 100 to 200 mg of vitamin B_6/d compared to those receiving a placebo. Another study observed that PMS symptoms improved with dietary modification and 250 mg/d of vitamin B_6/d.[54] However, the dangers of megadoses of vitamin B_6 have been documented. Schaumburg et al.[2] reported neurological disorders in subjects who self-prescribed large doses of vitamin B_6 to treat PMS symptoms. Thus, caution is indicated and indiscriminate use of vitamin B_6 is not advised.

E. FOLATE

Folate, also known as folic acid or folacin, is a B vitamin required for the synthesis of DNA, RNA, and protein. It helps vitamin B_{12} synthesize genetic material and form hemoglobin in red blood cells. A folate deficiency can impair cell division, leading to megaloblastic anemia, a type of anemia characterized by an increased level of megaloblasts, which are red blood cells much larger than the mature normal erythrocytes.

Folate status is currently a concern of health professionals because deficiency of this nutrient can lead to increased risk of neural tube defects.[55] Deficiencies of folate may result from: inadequate intake, impaired absorption, increased excretion, drug and alcohol abuse, cigarette smoking, and oral contraceptives.[55] Folate intake in the U.S. is low, particularly for females.[56] According to the Third National Health and Nutrition Examination Survey, the average folate intake of females between the ages of 12 and 79 ranged from 220 µg/d to 272 µg/d.[56] Female athletes, particularly young gymnasts and dancers, may also be at risk of folate deficiency.[12,43] Concerns about body weight, a lack of nutrition knowledge, and busy schedules are factors affecting nutrient intakes and food choices of these young athletes. Moffett[43] reported that folate intakes of high school gymnasts averaged 129 µg/d; candy, cakes, soda pop, and jellies contributed a good portion of the gymnasts' energy intake.

The RDA for females is 180 µg/d of folate, which is considerably lower than the 400 µg/d specified in the ninth edition of the RDAs. However, some scientists believe this amount is too low for women of childbearing age.[55] Studies have shown that folic acid supplementation prior to conception significantly reduced the risk of having an infant born with a neural tube defect.[55] An intake of 400 µg/d is considered necessary to maintain folate status and provide adequate protection.[55]

Folate is widely distributed in foods. Rich sources of folate include beef liver, orange juice, fresh spinach, and green leafy vegetables (Table 3.6). Fresh, uncooked fruits and vegetables are the best sources of folate because folate can easily be destroyed by heat during cooking.

Although folic acid is relatively nontoxic, supplementation may produce adverse effects in certain individuals.[57] Folic acid can interfere with the diagnosis and treatment of vitamin B_{12} deficiency in persons with pernicious anemia and may reduce the absorption of zinc.[58] Vitamin B_{12} status should be evaluated before initiating folate supplementation.[59]

F. VITAMIN B_{12}

Vitamin B_{12} (cyanocobalamin), plays an important role in folate metabolism. It is needed to convert folate coenzymes to their active forms which are required for normal DNA synthesis. Vitamin B_{12} is also essential for red blood cell formation as well as for proper nerve function, and for the maintenance and growth of the sheath that surrounds and protects nerve cells.

Absorption of vitamin B_{12} depends on the presence of an intrinsic factor, a protein-like compound produced by the lining of the stomach. Some individuals fail to excrete this intrinsic factor and as a result develop a B_{12} deficiency even though dietary intake is adequate.

The RDA for vitamin B_{12} for adults is 2.0 µg/d.[60] Vitamin B_{12} is found only in animal foods. The best sources of vitamin B_{12} are milk and milk products, beef, pork, eggs, and fish such as salmon and tuna. Fruits, vegetables, and grains contain virtually no vitamin B_{12}.

TABLE 3.6

Food Sources of Folate 🔖

RDA for women: 180 µg/d

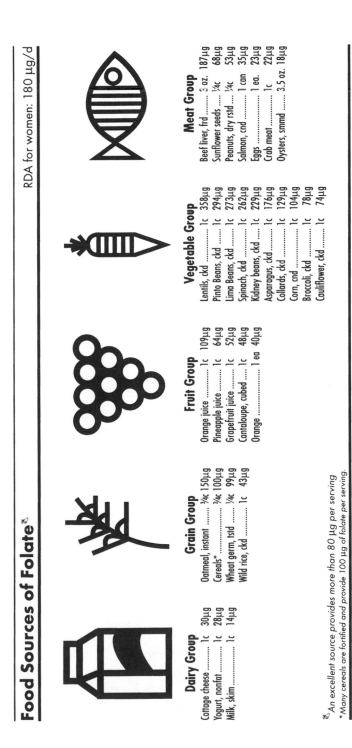

Dairy Group

Cottage cheese	1c	30µg
Yogurt, nonfat	1c	28µg
Milk, skim	1c	14µg

Grain Group

Oatmeal, instant	¾c	150µg
Cereals*	¾c	100µg
Wheat germ, tstd	¼c	99µg
Wild rice, ckd	1c	43µg

Fruit Group

Orange juice	1c	109µg
Pineapple juice	1c	64µg
Grapefruit juice	1c	52µg
Cantaloupe, cubed	1c	48µg
Orange	1 ea	40µg

Vegetable Group

Lentils, ckd	1c	358µg
Pinto Beans, ckd	1c	294µg
Lima Beans, ckd	1c	273µg
Spinach, ckd	1c	262µg
Kidney beans, ckd	1c	229µg
Asparagus, ckd	1c	176µg
Collards, ckd	1c	129µg
Corn, cnd	1c	104µg
Broccoli, ckd	1c	78µg
Cauliflower, ckd	1c	74µg

Meat Group

Beef liver, frd	3 oz.	187µg
Sunflower seeds	¼c	68µg
Peanuts, dry rstd	¼c	53µg
Salmon, cnd	1 can	35µg
Eggs	1 ea.	23µg
Crab meat	1c	22µg
Oysters, smmd	3.5 oz.	18µg

🔖 *An excellent source provides more than 80 µg per serving*

Many cereals are fortified and provide 100 µg of folate per serving.

Vitamin B_{12} deficiency is generally caused by malabsorption rather than inadequate dietary intake. Severe deficiency of this vitamin results in pernicious anemia, a condition in which the intrinsic factor is not produced, and thus vitamin B_{12} is not absorbed. Pernicious (deadly) anemia occurs primarily in older individuals and may be a genetic defect.[61] Characteristic symptoms include fatigue, weight loss, neurologic disturbances, and depression.

A dietary deficiency of vitamin B_{12} can occur in vegetarians who consume no animal products. Janelle and Barr[62] examined the nutrient intakes and eating behaviors of 23 vegetarian and 22 nonvegetarian women. Of the vegetarian women, 8 were vegans, 11 were lacto-ovovegetarians, and 4 were lactovegetarians. Results of their study revealed that vegetarianism was consistently associated with lower intakes of vitamin B_{12}, protein, cholesterol, and zinc. Compared to lacto-ovovegetarians, vegans had significantly lower ($P < 0.05$) mean intakes of vitamin B_{12}, 1.49 μg/d vs. 0.51 μg/d, respectively. Although a deficiency of vitamin B_{12} develops gradually over time, it can occur rapidly in breast-fed infants of vegan mothers.[63] Thus, it is important that vegans include a reliable source of vitamin B_{12} in the diet.[64] Vitamin B_{12} is available from vitamin supplements or fortified foods such as some breakfast cereals, soy beverages, and some brands of nutritional yeast.[64] Spirulina, seaweed, and tempeh were once thought to contain vitamin B_{12} in its active form; however, research has shown that as much as 80 to 94% of the vitamin B_{12} in these foods is inactive.[64]

1. The Role of Vitamin B_{12} in Exercise

One study has suggested that vitamin B_{12} metabolism may be altered in athletes during strenuous exercise. Singh et al.[65] studied the nutrient intake and biochemical status of ultramarathoners. Seventeen athletes (15 men and two women) recorded dietary data for 4 days and provided blood and urine samples. Mean intake of vitamin B_{12} from food alone was 6.1 μg/d and from food plus supplements, 51.3 μg/d. Despite a dietary intake well above recommended levels, blood concentrations of vitamin B_{12} (225.9 ± 27.3 pmol.l) were within the normal range (85 to 590 pmol.l). In an earlier study by Singh et al.,[66] blood levels of vitamin B_{12} increased significantly in response to vitamin mineral supplementation in male athletes. For this reason, Singh et al.[65] believe that ultramarathoners may have higher requirements for vitamin B_{12}. We await confirmation of this observation.

Many elite athletes take vitamin B_{12} supplements. Tour de France cyclists studied by Saris et al.[67] took several concentrated vitamin/mineral supplements, particularly vitamin B_{12} and iron. In another study,[68] vitamin B_{12} was listed as one of the 12 most popular supplements taken by triathletes. Although little is known about the rationales for supplement use among athletes, one would assume that the popularity of vitamin B_{12} is associated with increased performance capacity. However, few studies have reported on the effects of supplemental vitamin B_{12} on performance.

G. VITAMIN C

Few nutrients have attracted as much scientific and popular attention as vitamin C since the 1970s when Linus Pauling published *Vitamin C, the Common Cold and the Flu*. Pauling astonished the medical community by suggesting that daily doses of vitamin C in levels ranging from 1 to 2 g and even up to 10 g may help prevent colds.

Today, vitamin C's role as an antioxidant has again captured the attention of the scientific community. Like vitamin E, vitamin C may protect against cancer, heart disease, and cataracts.[69] It may also suppress harmful free radicals produced during exercise.[70]

Vitamin C exists in many forms. The two most active forms are L-ascorbic acid and L-dehydroascorbic acid.[71] While animals have the necessary enzymes to convert glucose or galactose into ascorbic acid, humans cannot synthesize vitamin C in the body and therefore must obtain it through food.

Vitamin C has a variety of roles:

- It is important in forming collagen, a protein that gives structure to bones, cartilage, muscle, and blood vessels.
- It helps to maintain capillaries, bones, and teeth.
- It facilitates the absorption of iron.
- It acts as an antioxidant.

The RDA for vitamin C is 60 mg a day.[72] During pregnancy and lactation, the RDA for vitamin C is increased to 70 mg/d and 95 mg/d, respectively. The primary sources of vitamin C are fruits and vegetables, especially citrus fruits. Foods that provide more than 30 mg per serving include strawberries, oranges, grapefruit, green peppers, broccoli, spinach, cauliflower, and brussel sprouts (Table 3.7). Most ready-to-eat cereals are fortified with vitamin C, and some fruit juices contain added vitamin C. However, not all juices and juice drinks contain the same amount of vitamin C. Many juice drinks contain less than 100% of the recommended daily value for vitamin C.

Vitamin C can be readily lost from foods during preparation, storage, or cooking. It is highly soluble in water and easily destroyed when exposed to air, heat, and alkali. To retain the vitamin C content of foods, serve fruits and vegetables raw whenever possible; steam, boil, or simmer foods in a minimal amount of water; cook potatoes in their skins; and store cut raw fruits and vegetables in an airtight container and refrigerate.

Certain population groups are at risk for vitamin C deficiency including smokers, the elderly, diabetics, and alcoholics.[73] Scurvy is the deficiency disease caused by a lack of vitamin C. Characteristic symptoms are a loss of appetite, anemia, poor wound healing, swollen and sore gums, bruising, tender joints, and reduced resistance to infection.

Because vitamin C is involved in wound healing, and because it is also a powerful antioxidant, an adequate dietary intake is important for athletes.

TABLE 3.7

Food Sources of Vitamin C ✿

RDA for women: 60 mg/d

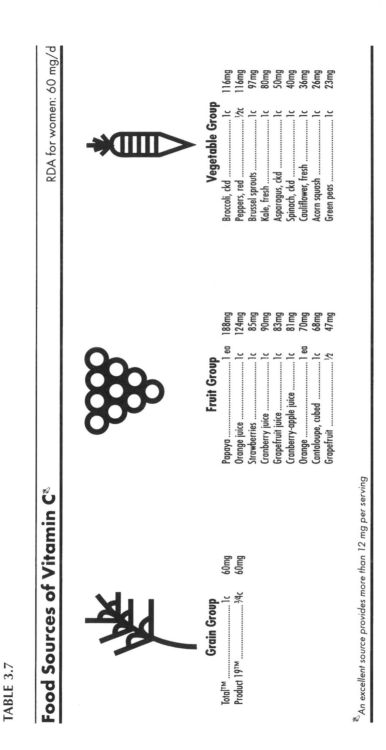

Grain Group

Total™	1c	60mg
Product 19™	3/4c	60mg

Fruit Group

Papaya	1 ea	188mg
Orange juice	1c	124mg
Strawberries	1c	85mg
Cranberry juice	1c	90mg
Grapefruit juice	1c	83mg
Cranberry-apple juice	1c	81mg
Orange	1 ea	70mg
Cantaloupe, cubed	1c	68mg
Grapefruit	1/2	47mg

Vegetable Group

Broccoli, ckd	1c	116mg
Peppers, red	1/2c	116mg
Brussel sprouts	1c	97mg
Kale, fresh	1c	80mg
Asparagus, ckd	1c	50mg
Spinach, ckd	1c	40mg
Cauliflower, fresh	1c	36mg
Acorn squash	1c	26mg
Green peas	1c	23mg

✿ An excellent source provides more than 12 mg per serving

Vitamin C deficiency may result in a wound with decreased tensile strength and decreased collagen synthesis.[74] Vitamin C may protect ligaments during healing so that a certain degree of strength can be regained.

Studies examining the nutrient intake of female athletes have generally reported dietary intakes of vitamin C greater than the RDA of 60 mg/d. Thus, compared to other nutrients, vitamin C is not a problem nutrient for female athletes in terms of deficiency. On the other hand, some groups of female athletes are heavy users of vitamin C supplements. Slavin et al.[75] reported elite female cyclists consumed megadoses (10 times the RDA) of vitamins, especially vitamin C and B-complex. Barr[76] also found that vitamin C supplements were frequently taken by female runners.

If dietary intake is adequate, will vitamin C supplements help improve performance? According to Gerster,[77] studies involving vitamin C supplementation have failed to show improvements in physical performance unless the subjects were deficient in vitamin C. There is some evidence that vitamin C supplementation may enhance resistance to upper respiratory tract infections in endurance athletes. Peters et al.[78] reported that symptoms of upper respiratory tract infections were significantly lower in runners consuming 600 mg/d of vitamin C before and after a 90 km race.

Because vitamin C is a water-soluble vitamin, it is generally considered safe. However, large doses (>500 mg/d) of vitamin C can be dangerous in some cases. For example, in the presence of high body iron stores, vitamin C becomes a very potent pro-oxidant.[79] According to Herbert,[79] about 10% of Americans are born with a gene for increased iron absorption (hemochromatosis) and 1% have iron overload. Men are more susceptible to iron overload than women and should be informed of the potential negative effects of excess vitamin C therapy.

Numerous studies are now underway using vitamin C and other antioxidants individually, in various combinations, or in combination with other nutrients to discover vitamins' ability to reduce the risk of chronic disease. Studies completed so far are encouraging, although conclusive data may not be available for years.

Until more information is available, athletes should consume a balanced diet that includes five servings of fruits and vegetables daily. If an athlete's diet is lacking in good sources of vitamin C, a multivitamin providing 250–500 mg/d appears to be safe.

IV. CONCLUSIONS

Dietary surveys have shown that diets of female athletes are low in several vitamins, which is most likely due to decreased energy intakes and inadequate food choices. Generally, it is agreed that exercise does not increase the requirement for most vitamins, and athletes who are consuming balanced diets do not need vitamin supplements.[80,81] However, some researchers[27] have suggested that thiamin requirements may be higher in athletes consuming high-calorie, high-carbohydrate diets. Additionally, the need for vitamin E may be increased in athletes exercising at high altitudes.[25]

Lawrence Machlin,[82] co-author of *Beyond Deficiency: New Views on the Function and Health Effects of Vitamins*, states that while traditionally nutritionists have been concerned with vitamins for their role in preventing vitamin-deficiency diseases, current research shows that some vitamins may have significant health effects beyond prevention of deficiency diseases. This may also be the case for vitamins and athletic performance. Scientists will continue to address two important questions: (1) does exercise increase the need for vitamins, and (2) will taking vitamin supplements improve performance?

REFERENCES

1. Belko, A. Z., Vitamins and exercise-an update, *Med. Sci. Sport Exerc.*, 19, S191, 1987.
2. Schaumburg, H., Kaplan, J., Windebank, A., Vick, N., Rasmus, S., Pleasure, D., and Brown, M. J., Sensory neuropathy from pyridoxine abuse, *N. Engl. J. Med.*, 309, 445, 1983.
3. McKenney, J. M., Proctor, J. D., Harris, S., and Chinchili, V. M., A comparison of the efficacy and toxic effects of sustained vs. immediate-release niacin in hypercholesterolemic patients, *J. Am. Med. Assoc.*, 271, 672, 1994.
4. Keith, R. E., Vitamins and physical performance, In *Nutrition in Exercise and Sport*, 2nd ed., Wolinsky, I. and Hickson, J. F., (Eds.) CRC Press, Inc., Boca Raton, 1994, 175.
5. Kanter, M. M., Nolte, L. A., and Hollosky, J. O., Effects of an antioxidant vitamin mixture on lipid peroxidation at rest and postexercise, *J. Appl. Physiol.*, 74, 965, 1993.
6. DeLuca, H. F., New concepts of vitamin D functions, In *Beyond Deficiency: New Views on the Function and Health Effects of Vitamins*, Sauberlich, H. E. and Machlin, L. J., (Eds.) *Ann. N.Y. Acad. Sci.*, New York, 669, 59, 1992.
7. Holick, M. F., McCollum Award Lecture, 1994: Vitamin D new horizons for the 21st century, *Am. J. Clin. Nutr.*, 60, 619, 1994.
8. Sills, I. N., Skuza, K. A., Horlick, M. N. B., Schwartz, M. S., and Rapaport, R., Vitamin D deficiency rickets, *Clin. Ped.*, August, 491, 1994.
9. Collins, E. D. and Norman, A. W., Vitamin D, In *Handbook of Vitamins*, 2nd ed., Machlin, L. J., (Ed.) Marcel Dekker, Inc., New York, 1991, 85.
10. Food and Nutrition Board, National Research Council, *Recommended Dietary Allowances*, 10th ed., National Academy Press, Washington, D.C., 1989, 95.
11. Lamar-Hildebrand, N., Saldanha, L., and Endres, J., Dietary and exercise practices of college-aged female bodybuilders, *J. Am. Diet. Assoc.*, 89, 1308, 1989.
12. Cohen, J. L., Potosnak, L., Frank, O., and Baker, H., A nutritional and hematologic assessment of elite ballet dancers, *Phys. Sportmed.*, 13, 43, 1985.
13. Bronner, F., Calcium and osteoporosis, *Am. J. Clin. Nutr.*, 60, 831, 1994.
14. Food and Nutrition Board, National Research Council, *Recommended Dietary Allowances*, 10th ed., National Academy Press, Washington, D.C., 1989, 97.
15. Collins, E. D. and Norman, A. W., Vitamin D, In *Handbook of Vitamins*, 2nd ed., Machlin, L. J., (Ed.) Marcel Dekker, Inc., New York, 1991, 89.
16. Packer, L., Protective role of vitamin E in biological systems, *Am. J. Clin. Nutr.*, 53, 1050S, 1991.
17. Keith, R. E., Vitamins and Physical Activity, In *Nutrition in Exercise and Sport*, 2nd ed., Wolinsky, I. and Hickson, J. F., (Eds.) CRC Press, Boca Raton, 1994, 177.
18. Machlin, L. J., Vitamin E, In *Handbook of Vitamins*, 2nd ed., Machlin, L. J., (Ed.) New York, 1991, 127.

19. Bendich, A. and Machlin, L. J., Safety of oral intake of vitamin E, *Am. J. Clin. Nutr.*, 48, 612, 1988.
20. Singh, V. N., A current perspective on nutrition and exercise, *J. Nutr.*, 122, 760, 1992.
21. Kagan, V. E., Spirichev, V. B., Serbinova, E. A., Witt, E., Erin, A. N., and Packer, L., The significance of vitamin E and free radicals in physical exercise, In *Nutrition in Exercise and Sport*, 2nd ed., Wolinsky, I. and Hickson, J. F., (Eds.) CRC Press, Boca Raton, 1994, 210.
22. Gillam, I., Skinner, S., and Telford, R., Effect of antioxidant supplements on indices of muscle damage and regeneration. *Med. Sci. Sports Exerc.*, 24, S17, 1992.
23. Simon-Schnass, I. M., Nutrition at high altitude, *J. Nutr.*, 122, 778, 1992.
24. Simon-Schnass, I. and Pabst, H., Influence of vitamin E on physical performance, *Int. J. Vit. Nutr. Res.*, 58, 49, 1988.
25. Simon-Schnass, I., Vitamin requirements for increased physical activity: vitamin E, In *Nutrition and Fitness for Athletes*, Simopoulous, A. P. and Pavlou, K. N., (Eds.), *World Rev. Nutr. Diet.*, Basel, Karger, 71, 144, 1993.
26. Sauberlich, H. E., Herman, Y. F., Stevens, C. O., and Herman, R. H., Thiamin requirements of the adult human, *Am. J. Clin. Nutr.*, 32, 2237, 1979.
27. van Erp Baart, A. M. J., Saris, W. H. M., Binkhorst, R. A., Vos, J. A., and Elvers, J. W. H., Nationwide survey on nutritional habits in elite athletes, Part II. Mineral and vitamin intake, *Int. J. Sports Med.*, 10, S11, 1989.
28. Food and Nutrition Board, National Research Council, *Recommended Dietary Allowances*, 10th ed., National Academy Press, Washington, D.C., 1989, 127.
29. Food and Nutrition Board, National Research Council, *Recommended Dietary Allowances*, 10th ed., National Academy Press, Washington, D.C., 1989, 133.
30. Kaiserauer, S., Synder, A. C., Sleeper, M., and Zierath, J., Nutritional, physiological, and menstrual status of distance runners, *Med. Sci. Sports Exerc.*, 21, 120, 1989.
31. Belko, A. Z., Obarzanek, E., Kalkwarf, H. J., Rotter, M. A., Bogusz, S., Miller, D., Haas, J. D., and Roe, D. A., Effects of exercise on riboflavin requirements of young women, *Am. J. Clin. Nutr.*, 37, 509, 1983.
32. Trebler Winters, L. R., Yoon, Jin-Sook, Kalkwarf, H. J., Davies, J. C., Berkowitz, M. G., Haas, J., and Roe, D. A., Riboflavin requirements and exercise adaptation in older women, *Am. J. Clin. Nutr.*, 56, 526, 1992.
33. Tremblay, A., Boilard, F., Breton, M. F., Bessette, H., and Roberge, A. G., The effects of riboflavin supplementation on the nutritional status and performance of elite swimmers, *Nutr. Res.*, 4, 201, 1984.
34. Keith, R. E. and Alt, L. A., Riboflavin status of female athletes consuming normal diets, *Nutr. Res.*, 11, 727, 1991.
35. Food and Nutrition Board, National Research Council, *Recommended Dietary Allowances*, 10th ed., National Academy Press, Washington, D.C., 1989, 139.
36. Alderman, J. D., Pasternak, R. C., Sacks, F. M., Smith, H. S., Monrad, E. S., and Grossman, W., Effect of a modified, well-tolerated niacin regimen on serum total cholesterol, high density lipoprotein cholesterol and the cholesterol to high density lipoprotein ratio, *Am. J. Cardiol.*, 64, 725, 1989.
37. Leklem, J. E., Vitamin B_6, In *Handbook of Vitamins*, 2nd ed., Machlin, L. J., (Ed.) Marcel Dekker, New York, 1991, 369.
38. Food and Nutrition Board, National Research Council, *Recommended Dietary Allowances*, 10th ed., National Academy Press, Washington, D.C., 1989, 144.
39. Kant, A. K. and Block, G., Dietary vitamin B-6 intake and food sources in the U.S. population: NHANES II, 1976-1980, *Am. J. Clin. Nutr.*, 52, 707, 1990.
40. Food and Nutrition Board, National Research Council, *Recommended Dietary Allowances*, 10th ed., National Academy Press, Washington, D.C., 1989, 143.
41. Manore, M. M., Besenfelder, P. D., Wells, C. L., Carroll, S. S., and Hooker, S. P., Nutrient intakes and iron status in female long-distance runners during training, *J. Am. Diet. Assoc.*, 89, 257, 1989.

42. Keith, R. E., O'Keeffe, K. A., Alt, L. A., and Young, K. L., Dietary status of trained female cyclists, *J. Am. Diet. Assoc.*, 89, 1620, 1989.
43. Moffatt, R. J., Dietary status of elite female high school gymnasts: Inadequacy of vitamin and mineral intake, *J. Am. Diet. Assoc.*, 84, 1361, 1984.
44. Hickson, J. F., Schrader, J., and Trischler, L. C., Dietary intakes of female basketball and gymnastics athletes, *J. Am. Diet. Assoc.*, 86, 251, 1986.
45. Rucinski, A., Relationship of body image and dietary intake of competitive ice skaters, *J. Am. Diet. Assoc.*, 89, 98, 1989.
46. Bergen-Cico, D. K. and Short, S. H., Dietary intakes, energy expenditures, and anthropometric characteristics of adolescent female cross-country runners, *J. Am. Diet. Assoc.*, 92, 611, 1992.
47. Rokitzki, L., Sagredos, A. N., Reub, F., Cufi, D., and Keul, J., Assessment of vitamin B_6 status of strength and speedpower athletes, *J. Am. Coll. Nutr.*, 13, 87, 1994.
48. Manore, M. M., Vitamin B_6 and exercise, *Int. J. Sport Nutr.*, 4, 89, 1994.
49. Manore, M. M., Leklem, J. E., and Walter, M. C., Vitamin B-6 metabolism as affected by exercise in trained and untrained women fed diets differing in carbohydrate and vitamin B-6 content, *Am. J. Clin. Nutr.*, 46, 995, 1987.
50. Crozier, P. G., Cordain, L., and Sampson, D. A., Exercise-induced changes in plasma vitamin B-6 concentrations do not vary with exercise intensity, *Am. J. Clin. Nutr.*, 60, 552, 1994.
51. Rose, D. P., The interactions between vitamin B_6 and hormones, *Vitam. Horm.*, 36, 53, 1978.
52. Abraham, G. E., Premenstrual tension, *Curr. Prob. Obstet. Gynecol. Fertil.*, 3, 1, 1980.
53. Williams, M. J., Harris, R. I., and Dean, R. C., Controlled trial of pyridoxine in the premenstrual syndrome, *J. Int. Med. Res.*, 13, 174, 1985.
54. Berman, M. K., Taylor, M. L., and Freeman, E., Vitamin B_6 in premenstrual syndrome, *J. Am. Diet. Assoc.*, 90, 859, 1990.
55. Picciano, M. F., Green, T., and O'Connor, D. L., The folate status of women and health, *Nutr. Today*, 29, 20, 1994.
56. Alaimo, K., McDowell, M. A., Briefel, R. R., Bischof, A. M., Caughman, C. R., Loria, C. M., and Johnson, C. L., Dietary intake of vitamins, minerals, and fiber of persons ages 2 months and over in the United States:Third National Health and Nutrition Examination Survey, Phase I, 1988-91, Advance data from vital and health statistics; no 258. Hyattsville, Maryland: National Center for Health Statistics, 1994.
57. Zimmermann, M. B. and Shane, B., Supplemental folic acid, *Am. J. Clin. Nutr.*, 58, 127, 1993.
58. Butterworth, C. E. and Tamura, T., Folic acid safety and toxicity: a brief review, *Am. J. Clin. Nutr.*, 50, 353, 1989.
59. Bailey, L. B., Evaluation of a new Recommended Dietary Allowance for folate, *J. Am. Diet. Assoc.*, 92, 463, 1992.
60. Food and Nutrition Board, National Research Council, *Recommended Dietary Allowance*, 10th ed., National Academy Press, Washington, D.C., 1989, 152.
61. Ellenbogen, L. and Cooper, B. A., Vitamin B_{12} In *Handbook of Vitamins*, Machlin, L. J. (Ed.), Marcel Dekker, Inc., New York, 1991, 491.
62. Janelle, K. C. and Barr, S. I., Nutrient intakes and eating behavior scores of vegetarian and nonvegetarian women, *J. Am. Diet. Assoc.*, 95, 180, 1995.
63. Graham, S. M., Arvela, O. M., and Wise, G. A., Long-term neurologic consequences of nutritional vitamin B_{12} deficiency in infants, *J. Pediatr.*, 121, 710, 1992.
64. Position of The American Dietetic Association: vegetarian diets. *J. Am. Diet. Assoc.*, 93, 1317, 1993.
65. Singh, A., Evans, P., Gallagher, K. L., and Deuster, P. A., Dietary intakes and biochemical profiles of nutritional status of ultramarathoners, *Med. Sci. Sports Exerc.*, 25, 328, 1993.
66. Singh, A., Moses, F. M., and Deuster, P. A., Vitamin and mineral status in physically active men: effects of a high-potency supplement, *Am. J. Clin. Nutr.*, 55, 1, 1992.

67. Saris, W. H. M., van Erp-Baart, M. A., Brouns, F., Westerterp, K. R., and ten Hoor, F., Study on food intake and energy expenditure during extreme sustained exercise: The Tour de France. *Int. J. Sports Med.*, 10, S26, 1989.
68. Khoo, Chor-San, Rawson, N. E., Robinson, M. L., and Stevenson, R. J., Nutrient intake and eating habits of triathletes, *Ann. Sports Med.*, 3, 144, 1987.
69. Block, G. and Langseth, L., Antioxidant vitamins and disease prevention, *Food Technol.*, July, 80, 1994.
70. Jenkins, R. R., Exercise, oxidative stress, and antioxidants: A review, *Int. J. Sport. Nutr.*, 3, 356, 1993.
71. Moser, U. and Bendich, A., Vitamin C, In *Handbook of Vitamins*, Machlin, L. J. (Ed.), Marcel Dekker, Inc., New York, 1991, 198.
72. Food and Nutrition Board, National Research Council, *Recommended Dietary Allowance*, 10th ed., National Academy Press, Washington, D.C., 1989, 117.
73. Moser, U. and Bendich, A., Vitamin C, In *Handbook of Vitamins*, Machlin, L. J., (Ed.), Marcel Dekker, Inc., New York, 1991, 204.
74. Stanish, W. D., O'Grady, P., and Dillon, J. E., Knee ligament sprains — acute and chronic, In *Oxford Textbook of Sports Medicine*, Harries, M., Williams, C., Stanish, W. D., and Micheli, L. J. (Eds.), Oxford University Press, New York, 1994, 365.
75. Slavin, J. L. and McNamara, E. A., Nutritional practices of women cyclists, including recreational riders and elite racers, In *Sport, Health and Nutrition*, Vol. 2, Human Kinetics Publishing, Champaign, IL, 1986.
76. Barr, S. I., Nutrition knowledge and selected nutritional practices of female recreational athletes, *J. Nutr. Educ.*, 18, 167, 1986.
77. Gerster, H., The role of vitamin C in athletic performance, *J. Am. Coll. Nutr.*, 8, 636, 1989.
78. Peters, E. M., Goetzsche, J. M., Grobbelaar, B., and Noakes, T. D., Vitamin C supplementation reduces the incidence of postrace symptoms of upper-respiratory-tract infection in ultramarathon runners, *Am. J. Clin. Nutr.*, 57, 170, 1993.
79. Herbert, V., Viewpoint: Does mega-C do more good than harm, or more harm than good?, *Nutr. Today*, February, 28, 1993.
80. Singh, A., Moses, F. M., and Deuster, P. A. Chronic multivitamin-mineral supplementation does not enhance physical performance, *Med. Sci. Sports Exerc.*, 24, 726, 1992.
81. Weight, L. M., Noakes, T. D., Labadarios, D., Graves, J., Jacobs, P., and Berman, P. A., Vitamin and mineral status of trained athletes including the effects of supplementation, *Am. J. Clin. Nutr.*, 47, 186, 1988.
82. Sauberlich, H. E. and Machlin, L. J. In *Beyond Deficiency: New Views on the Function and Health Effects of Vitamins*, Annals of the New York Academy of Sciences, 699, 1, 1992.

Chapter 4

THE MINERALS: CALCIUM, IRON, AND ZINC

CONTENTS

I. INTRODUCTION

Minerals are inorganic elements, of which 17 are known to be essential in human nutrition. The major minerals — calcium, sodium, potassium, chlorine, magnesium, phosphorus, and sulfur — are required in relatively large quantities in the body. The remaining minerals are referred to as trace or minor minerals because they are needed only in small amounts. The trace minerals include iron, zinc, selenium, chromium, fluoride, iodine, and copper.

Like vitamins, minerals have specific functions in the body. They help maintain normal functioning of muscle and nerve tissue, blood clotting, body fluid balance, and bone formation. Minerals are also components of enzymes involved in the regulation of metabolism. A summary of the minerals is provided in Table 4.1.

The body's ability to absorb and utilize minerals is affected by the presence of other nutrients and dietary substances. For example, vitamin D improves calcium absorption and vitamin C enhances iron absorption, while excess zinc can interfere with the metabolism of iron and copper.

As shown in Chapter 1, Table 1.4, studies of female athletes have reported low dietary intakes of several minerals, specifically the major mineral calcium and the trace minerals iron and zinc. This chapter highlights the functions of these three minerals, their distribution in foods, recommended amounts, effects of deficiency and or toxicity, and their role in exercise.

II. CALCIUM

A. ROLE OF CALCIUM

Calcium, an essential nutrient, is needed for bone development and maintenance. The adult human body contains about 1200 g of calcium. Of this, 99% is deposited in the bones and teeth. The other 1% is found in blood and extracellular fluids and is responsible for maintaining normal heartbeat and muscle contractions and for enzyme activity. These calcium-related functions are regulated by three hormones: parathyroid hormone, calcitonin, and calcitrol, an active metabolite of vitamin D. Together, these hormones maintain calcium metabolism.

Calcium deserves special attention because of its role in bone health and osteoporosis. It has also been shown to protect against hypertension and certain cancers.[1] Calcium is of particular concern among women because many do not consume adequate amounts of this mineral. The RDA for calcium is 800 mg/d for children and adults and 1200 mg/d for adolescent, pregnant, and lactating women.[2] Data from the USDA 1987–1988 Nationwide Food Consumption Survey reported a mean calcium intake of 789 mg/d for females ages 12–19, 630 mg/d for women ages 20–29, and less than 600 mg/d for women ages 30–69.[3] In another survey, Chapman et al.[4] reported that over 40% of

TABLE 4.1 The Minerals

Nutrient	Functions	Sources	RDA[a]
Calcium	Aids in formation and maintenance of strong bones and teeth. Permits healthy nerve functioning and normal blood clotting	Yogurt, milk, cheese, salmon, green leafy vegetables	1,200 mg
Phosphorus	Aids in formation and maintenance of strong bones and teeth. Part of cell membrane and ATP	Meat, fish, poultry, dairy products, whole grains	1,200 mg
Magnesium	Aids in bone structure, nerve impulse transmission, and protein formation	Vegetables, beans, nuts, milk, fruit	280 mg
Iron	Helps build red blood cells which carry oxygen to all parts of the body	Red meats, fish, poultry, eggs, legumes, shellfish, dried fruit	15 mg
Potassium	Electrolyte; maintains fluid and electrolyte balance and muscle contraction	Fruits, vegetables, grains, meats, and milk	2,000 mg[b]
Sodium	Electrolyte; maintains normal fluid balance and nerve impulse transmission	Salt, soy sauce, processed foods	500 mg[b] 2,400 mg[c]
Chloride	Electrolyte; part of hydrochloric acid in the stomach	Salt, soy sauce, water	750 mg[b]
Sulfur	A part of certain amino acids, the vitamins biotin and thiamin, and the hormone insulin	Eggs, meat, fish and poultry, dairy products	No RDA
Iodine	A component of the thyroid hormone thyroxine, which regulates growth and development; basal metabolic rate	Iodized salt, seafood, bread, grains	150 µg
Zinc	Plays a role in the formation of genetic material and proteins; wound healing, immune system, and normal sexual growth and development	Red meats, fish, shellfish, poultry, vegetables, grains	12 mg
Selenium	Antioxidant; works with vitamin E	Seafoods, organ meats, grains, and some vegetables depending on soil	55 µg

[a] Except where indicated all RDAs reflect daily amounts established for 19–24 year-old females.
[b] Minimum daily requirement for healthy persons.
[c] Recommended daily intake.

women between the ages of 22 and 85 years had calcium intakes below 60% of the RDA.

Low calcium intakes have also been reported among many female athletes, including gymnasts, runners, cyclists, swimmers, field athletes, dancers, and bodybuilders (Table 1.4). Elite female athletes studied by Grandjean et al.[5] had a mean calcium intake of 981 mg/d, which for all subjects combined represented 92% of the RDA. However, of the 54 female athletes 19 years and older, 26% had calcium intakes less than 70% of the RDA, while 55% of the female athletes 18 years and under consumed less than 70% of the RDA. Webster and Barr[6] studied calcium intakes of female gymnasts and speed skaters and reported that despite mean dietary calcium intakes above the RDA, individual calcium intakes were low.

Diets low in milk and dairy products or diets low in total calories are contributing factors of inadequate calcium intakes. A diet that consistently excludes or limits dairy products will not only supply less calcium, but may also limit other essential nutrients such as riboflavin, vitamin D, protein, phosphorus, and vitamin A found in foods containing calcium.[7]

Chapman et al.[4] examined knowledge, attitudes, and behaviors influencing the calcium intake of women. Their study reported several important conclusions: 25% of the women who had low calcium intakes of less than 60% of the RDA were not aware their dietary intakes of calcium were low. Almost half (46%) of the women could not name nondairy food sources of calcium. One third of the women surveyed believed that dairy products were high in calories and cholesterol; 12% of the the the women avoided milk because of problems with digestion.

Many female athletes avoid milk and dairy foods because they believe these foods are high in fat and calories. However, a recent study[7] demonstrated that it is possible to consume increased amounts of calcium without drastically changing total fat intake. Subjects were divided into three groups: (1) a diet group, counseled to increase calcium intake to 1500 mg/d through foods, (2) a supplemental group, (1000 mg/d calcium carbonate), or (3) a placebo group. Results showed that over a 12-week period, 83% of the subjects in the diet group achieved the goal of 1500 mg/d of calcium by eating proportionately higher amounts of yogurt, as well as skim and 1% low-fat milk. The average total fat intake of female subjects in the diet group was 66 g/d at baseline and 69 g/d during the study period. The subjects in the diet group received dietary information on how to maintain a high-calcium diet demonstrating that nutrition education can produce positive changes in short-term eating behavior.

B. FOOD SOURCES

Although calcium is widely distributed in plant and animal foods, dairy products are the richest source of calcium. Over 50% of the calcium in the typical American diet comes from milk and milk products including yogurt, cheese, and milk-based desserts such as ice cream and puddings.[3] Milk and cheese used as ingredients in meat, grain, and vegetable dishes also contribute about 20% of calcium in the diet. Other good sources of calcium include some green vegetables such as turnip greens, broccoli, and okra, and fish with small bones, such as salmon and sardines (Table 4.2). Tofu and calcium-fortified soy milk are important sources of calcium in diets of vegans.[8]

TABLE 4.2

Food Sources of Calcium 🐝

RDA for women: 1200 mg/d

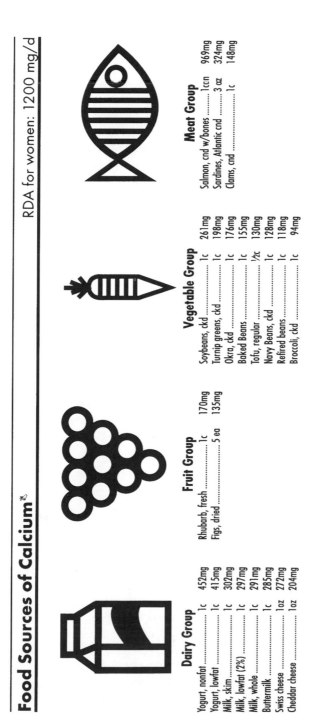

Dairy Group

Yogurt, nonfat 1c	452mg
Yogurt, lowfat 1c	415mg
Milk, skim 1c	302mg
Milk, lowfat (2%) 1c	297mg
Milk, whole 1c	291mg
Buttermilk 1c	285mg
Swiss cheese 1oz	272mg
Cheddar cheese 1oz	204mg

Fruit Group

Rhubarb, fresh 1c	170mg
Figs, dried ....5 ea	135mg

Vegetable Group

Soybeans, ckd 1c	261mg
Turnip greens, ckd 1c	198mg
Okra, ckd 1c	176mg
Baked Beans 1c	155mg
Tofu, regular ....½c	130mg
Navy Beans, ckd 1c	128mg
Refried beans 1c	118mg
Broccoli, ckd 1c	94mg

Meat Group

Salmon, cnd w/bones 1ccn	969mg
Sardines, Atlantic cnd ....3 oz	324mg
Clams, cnd 1c	148mg

🐝*An excellent source provides more than 200 mg per serving*

C. CALCIUM REQUIREMENTS AND RECOMMENDED AMOUNTS

In 1994, a National Institutes of Health (NIH) Consensus Development Conference brought together experts from a variety of health fields to review studies related to calcium intake and its effect on calcium balance, bone mass, and the prevention of osteoporosis.[9,10] The purpose of the conferences was to address three major questions: (1) What is the optimal amount of calcium intake? (2) What are the important factors for achieving optimal calcium intake?, and (3) What are the best ways to attain optimal calcium intake? Based on their results, the panel concluded that the calcium intake for most age groups should be greater than the Recommended Dietary Allowances (Table 4.3).

TABLE 4.3   National Institutes of Health's Optimal Calcium Requirements

Group	Optimal Daily Intake (mg of calcium)
Infants	
Birth–6 months	400
6 months–1 year	600
Children	
1–5 years	800
6–10 years	800–1,200
Adolescents/Young Adults	
11–24 years	1,200–1,500
Women	
25–65 years	1,000
Over 50 years (postmenopausal)	
On estrogens	1,000
Not on estrogens	1,500
Over 65 years	1,500
Pregnant and nursing	1,200–1,500

From *Optimal Calcium Intake, NIH Consensus Statement,* 1994, June 6; 12(4): 1–31.

1. Adolescent Female

Three major studies support higher calcium intakes during childhood.[11-13] Matkovic et al.[11] evaluated the influence of calcium intake and heredity on bone mass in adolescent females and concluded that a calcium intake of up to 1800 mg/d may be necessary to attain optimal peak bone mass.

Abrams and Stuff[12] examined the effects of self-selected diets on calcium absorption and retention in 51 girls during pre-, early, and late puberty. Results of their study showed that mean calcium intakes were below the RDA of 1200 mg/d. The early pubertal period was associated with higher dietary calcium absorption (34%) than prepubertal (27%) or late pubertal periods (25%). Calculated calcium retention averaged 132 mg/d in prepubertal girls, 161 mg/d in early pubertal girls, and 44 mg/d in late pubertal girls. The investigators concluded that the current calcium intake of girls during the pubertal growth period is not sufficient for maximum calcium retention.

Lee et al.[13] studied the effects of calcium supplementation on bone mineral acquisition in children on low-calcium diets (<300 mg/d). Children were randomly assigned to either a supplemental group (300 mg/d calcium carbonate) or a placebo group. Bone mineral content (BMC) was measured before the study, and after 6, 12, and 18 months of supplementation, by single-photon absorptometry. After 18 months, the supplemental group had significantly greater gains in radial BMC compared to the placebo group.

Andon et al.[14] reviewed the literature and concluded that the RDAs are not adequate to support optimal bone mass gain during growth and development. Based on intervention trials with calcium supplementation, recommendations are made for an RDA of 1250 mg/d during childhood and 1450 mg/d during adolescence. These levels agree with threshold intakes determined by Matkovic and Heaney.[15] Threshold intakes are values which provide sufficient calcium to ensure maximal skeletal retention of calcium.[15] Present data show that above this threshold there is no further increase in skeletal retention of calcium and urinary calcium will begin to increase more rapidly.[16]

2. Adult Female

During the adult years, calcium intake should be sufficient to preserve calcium balance and to maintain an intact skeleton.[11] After age 35, resorption rates increase, and bone mass declines with the decrease in estrogen production associated with the onset of menopause. However, data show that consuming more than 800 mg/d of calcium during adulthood helps decrease the rate of bone loss and maximize the potential for maintaining optimal peak bone mass in premenopausal women.[17,18]

Although estrogen replacement therapy is currently the most effective way to protect bones during postmenopausal years, data have shown beneficial effects of increased calcium and vitamin D intake on bone health in middle-aged and elderly women. Hu et al.[19] compared calcium intake and bone density in 843 Chinese women 35 to 75 years of age from five rural counties where calcium intakes varied greatly, from 230 mg/d to 724 mg/d. Results showed higher bone densities of the distal and midradius among women in rural counties with higher calcium intakes.

3. Elderly Female

Two studies using calcium supplements showed a decrease in the incidence of fractures among elderly women.[20,21] In a study by Chapuy et al.,[20] hip fracture rates decreased by 43% in elderly women receiving calcium (1200 mg/d) and vitamin D supplements (200 IU/d) compared to a placebo group. In another study, Reid et al.[21] reported significantly fewer fractures in women receiving calcium supplementation (1000 mg/d) for 4 years.

These studies demonstrate that calcium and vitamin D are important for bone health in postmenopausal women. Yet national surveys have shown that in women over age 50, calcium intakes below 800 mg/d are common[3] and often accompanied by inadequate intake of vitamin D. The NIH consensus panel recommends that all adults over age 65 should have calcium intakes of 1500 mg/d.[9]

D. CALCIUM ABSORPTION

Absorbability of calcium is an important consideration in ensuring adequate calcium status. The body's ability to absorb dietary calcium is affected by the presence of other nutrients and dietary substances as well as physiological factors. Factors which increase calcium absorption include:

Physiological need. Calcium absorption increases during times of increased need, such as during the adolescent growth spurt or pregnancy and lactation, and it declines with age. Adolescent females absorb more calcium and excrete less calcium than do adult females with the same calcium intakes.[22]

Vitamin D. Vitamin D is necessary for increasing the efficiency of calcium absorption, particularly when calcium intake is low. In the absence of vitamin D, less than 10% of dietary calcium may be aborbed.[9]

Phosphorus. Phosphorus makes up about half the weight of bone mineral and thus must be present in adequate amounts in the diet to maintain the skeleton.

Estrogen. Estrogen protects bone by increasing the absorption of calcium and its uptake into the bone.

Physical Exercise. Exercise can result in increased bone mass, a slowing of bone loss, and an increase in bone mineral content.

Urinary calcium excretion is an important determinant of calcium retention. Several dietary factors are known to influence urinary calcium excretion, including sodium, protein, and caffeine. According to Matkovic et al.,[16] sodium is one of the most important determinants of urinary calcium excretion. They measured the effects of various nutrients on urinary calcium excretion of young females, aged 8 to 13 years and found a negative association between urinary calcium excretion and bone mass, with sodium being one of the most important determinants of urinary calcium excretion. Matkovic's study[16] has important implications for nutrition educators studying eating patterns and food choices of young adolescent girls. Young girls consuming low-calcium, high-sodium diets may be at risk for reduced bone mineral density. As such, nutrition messages designed to increase calcium awareness and intakes of young women should include information about sodium in the diet.

There is also a positive relationship between dietary protein and urinary calcium excretion. High protein intakes increase calcium excretion[23] and have been negatively associated with bone mineral content in premenopausal women.[24]

Additionally, caffeine has been shown to increase urinary calcium excretion.[25] High caffeine intakes may compromise bone health when coupled with a low calcium intake.[26] A recent study[27] concluded that consuming caffeine in amounts equal to or greater than 2 to 3 cups/d of brewed coffee may accelerate bone loss in women with calcium intakes below the RDA. Another study[28] involving premenopausal vegetarian and nonvegetarian women consuming 972 mg/d and 770 mg/d of calcium, respectively, reported that high caffeine intake led to higher urinary calcium excretion, but no correlation was found between bone density and caffeine intake.

Two inhibitors of calcium absorption found in plant foods are oxalate and phytate. Oxalate, which is found in high amounts in spinach, dry beans, and rhubarb, is the strongest inhibitor of calcium absorption. Phytate, a storage form of phosphorus in plants, reduces the bioavailability of calcium but to a smaller degree than oxalate.[29] Heaney et al.[30] reported that absorption of calcium from spinach was 5% compared to 27.6% from milk. In contrast, the absorption of calcium from low-oxalate vegetables such as kale and broccoli, is excellent, even higher than milk[31] (Table 4.4). The bioavailability of calcium from soybeans, which contain both phytate and oxalate, is also good.[29] Of substances tested to date, only wheat bran has been shown to decrease the absorption of calcium.[32]

E. OSTEOPOROSIS

Osteoporosis is a disease characterized by low bone mass, deterioration of bone tissue leading to enhanced bone fragility, and increased risk of fracture.[33] It is a major public health problem in the U.S., affecting 26 million white women annually.[34] Approximately 1.7 million hip fractures occurred in 1990 throughout the world.[35] Total fracture costs each year in the U.S. alone are more than 10 billion dollars.[36] Fracture risk is influenced by genetic, endocrine, and lifestyle factors. Of all diseases, osteoporosis is most linked to women because (1) women have 15% lower bone mineral density and 30% less bone mass than men, (2) the rate of bone mass declines rapidly after the onset of natural or induced menopause, and (3) because more women than men consume diets low in calcium.[26]

The relationship between calcium and osteoporosis has been explored for many years. At one time, scientists believed that the body could adapt to relatively low calcium intakes.[37] But subsequent research by Heaney et al.[38] showed that inadequate calcium intake during childhood and adolescence could result in debilitating bone loss later in life. More recent observations further demonstrate that high intakes of calcium and vitamin D contribute to optimal bone mass development.[1] For women, an adequate intake of calcium between menarch and late adolescence is thought to play a critical role in reducing the risk of osteoporosis.[26]

It is well known that the poorest absorption of calcium occurs in women with low estrogen levels. Estrogen deficiency is the major cause of bone loss

TABLE 4.4   Food Sources of Bioavailable Calcium

Food[a]	Serving size g	Calcium content mg	Fractional absorption %	Estimated absorbable Ca/serving mg	Servings needed to = 240 mL milk n
Milk	240	300	32.1	96.3	1
Almonds, dry roasted	28	80	21.2	17.0	5.7
Beans, pinto	86	44.7	17.0	7.6	12.7
Beans, red	172	40.5	17.0	6.9	14
Beans, white	110	113	17.0	19.2	5
Broccoli	71	35	52.6	18.4	5.2
Brussel sprouts	78	19	63.8	12.1	8
Cabbage, Chinese	85	79	53.8	42.5	2.3
Cabbage, green	75	25	64.9	16.2	5.9
Cauliflower	62	17	68.6	11.7	8.2
Citrus punch with CCM	240	300	50.0	150.0	0.64
Fruit punch with CCM	240	300	52.0	156.0	0.62
Kale	65	47	58.8	27.6	3.5
Kohlrabi	82	20	67.0	13.4	7.2
Mustard greens	72	64	57.8	37.0	2.6
Radish	50	14	74.4	10.4	9.2
Rutabaga	85	36	61.4	22.1	4.4
Sesame seeds, no hulls	28	37	20.8	7.7	12.2
Soy milk	120	5	31.0	1.6	60.4
Spinach	90	122	5.1	6.2	15.5
Tofu, calcium set	126	258	31.0	80.0	1.2
Turnip greens	72	99	51.6	51.1	1.9
Watercress	17	20	67.0	13.4	7.2

a   Based on 1/2-cup serving size except for milk, citrus punch, and fruit juice (1 cup) and
      almonds and sesame seeds (1 oz.).

From Weaver, C. M. and Plawecki, K. L., Dietary calcium adequacy of a vegetarian diet ©*Am.
J. Clin. Nutr.,* 1994, 59 (suppl) 1238S–1241S. With permission.

for the first two decades following natural menopause.[39] Estrogen affects both
the absorption and excretion of calcium. In the absence of estrogen, a women
absorbs calcium less efficiently and excretes it more vigorously.[40]

Estrogen replacement therapy greatly reduces the risk of osteoporotic
fractures by increasing the absorption of calcium and its uptake and deposition
into bone.[26] Initiated at the onset of menopause, estrogen therapy can decrease
the incidence of osteoporosis-related fractures by about 50%.[26] The effects of
estrogen last for as long as therapy continues; bone loss will recur if estrogen
therapy is discontinued.[33]

F.   EXERCISE AND BONE DENSITY

Exercise helps minimize bone loss in women.[17,24,41,42] Although the type,
intensity, and duration of exercise necessary to influence bone mass has not

been determined, it is generally accepted that regular weight-bearing activity slows the rate of bone loss and strengthens existing bone.

Research linking regular physical exercise and increased bone density comes from studies conducted with athletes.[43] More than 20 years ago, Nilsson and Westlin[44] reported that athletes from various sports had greater bone mineral density than nonathletes. Their study also found differences within sport groups suggesting that bone hypertrophy is specific to the amount and type of stress placed on the bone. Weightlifters had the greatest bone mass, followed by throwers, runners, and soccer players. Swimmers had the least bone mass.

A more recent study suggests that bone mineral content is increased by resistence training. Heinrich et al.[45] compared the bone mineral content of cyclically menstruating female bodybuilders, swimmers, runners, and controls. Results of their study showed that the average bone mineral content of the bodybuilders was greater than the bone mineral content of swimmers, runners, or nonathletes. However, as previously indicated, many factors influence bone mineral content, including calcium, sodium, and protein as well as total energy intake. Furthermore, estrogen has a direct effect on bone mineral density. Hypoestrogenism can reduce peak bone mass and increase an athlete's risk of stress fractures and premature osteoporosis.

G. AMENORRHEA AND EXERCISE

In 1991, the American College of Sports Medicine established a task force on women's issues in sports to address an area of growing concern in sports medicine: a triad of disorders observed in adolescent and young female athletes.[46] This triad includes three major health problems: amenorrhea, eating disorders, and osteoporosis (Figure 4.1).

Some groups of female athletes, such as runners, gymnasts, and dancers, exercise and diet to the point where they develop eating problems and menstrual irregularities. Amenorrhea, the absence of menstrual cycles, is characterized by low levels of circulating estrogen.[47] Estrogen-deficient athletes risk reduced bone mineral content and bone density.[48,49]

There are two major categories of amenorrhea: primary and secondary.[50] Primary amenorrhea is the absence of menstrual periods by age 16. Secondary amenorrhea is the absence of three to six consecutive menstrual periods after normal menarche has occurred.

Many nutritional and physiological factors have been associated with amenorrhea. Frequently cited are low calorie intake, low body weight, eating disorders, low percent body fat, excessive exercise, delayed menarche, stress, and decreased gonadotropin secretion.[51-56] According to Putukian[50] exercise-associated amenorrhea is the most frequent cause of amenorrhea in athletes, and it is considered a hypothalamic disorder.

In athletes, the prevalence of amenorrhea varies among sport groups. In a study of 226 elite athletes, gymnasts had the highest incidence of amenorrhea

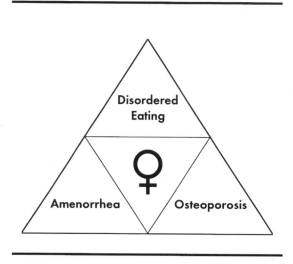

FIGURE 4.1   The Female Athlete Triad.

(71%), followed by lightweight rowers (46%) and runners (45%).[52] In ballet dancers, the reported incidence of amenorrhea ranges from 27 to 47%.[52,57]

The primary health concern of amenorrheic athletes has been infertility. However, research has shown that one of the long-term consequences of exercise-induced amenorrhea is premature osteoporosis.[56] Compared to regularly menstruating women, amenorrheic athletes have lower bone mineral content of the lumbar spine.[47,58,59] Some data have also found a greater incidence of scoliosis (curvature of the spine) and stress fractures in amenorrheic athletes.[55,60-62]

In addition to the absence of menstrual periods, infrequent periods can influence bone health. This condition, known as oligomenorrhea, is defined as three to six menstrual cycles a year at intervals greater than 36 days.[50] Micklesfield et al.[49] reported in premenopausal ultramarathon runners, a history of oligomenorrhea was significantly related to reduced lumbar spine bone mineral density.

The primary cause for reduced bone mineral density in amenorrheic athletes is low circulating levels of estrogens (estradiol and estrone).[56,63,64] Secondary causes include nutritional factors such as low body weight, low percent body fat, eating disorders, low calorie intake, and low calcium intake.[65]

In managing exercise-associated amenorrhea, professionals should encourage athletes to resume their periods by training less intensely.[61] Although some data show that increases in bone density may occur before the return of normal menses,[64] these increases still may be significantly below the normal range for optimal bone health.

Secondly, it is recommended that athletes gain weight (if they are underweight) and improve their eating habits. To attain optimal calcium intake levels, an increased consumption of dairy products and/or calcium-rich vegetables is advised. Studies comparing the diets of regularly menstruating athletes to amenorrheic athletes indicate that amenorrheic athletes tend to eat fewer calories[47,53] and have lower fat intakes,[47,62,63,66] both of which may negatively affect calcium intake.

Coaches, trainers, physicians, and sport nutritionists should educate athletes about long-term risks associated with amenorrhea and/or oligomenorrhea, emphasizing the adverse effects on bone health and athletic performance. If female athletes are not willing to change their training routine or diet, estrogen replacement therapy and calcium supplementation may be necessary to preserve and protect bone mass.[50,65]

H. CALCIUM SUPPLEMENTATION

Although the effectiveness of calcium supplements in preventing bone loss has not been proven definitively, more and more female athletes are taking them.[67] Pate et al.[68] reported that 49% of women runners used calcium supplements. In another study,[69] 33% of recreational runners reported taking calcium supplements.

There are more than a dozen commonly prescribed calcium supplements available today.[70] Calcium carbonate is frequently recommended because of its high calcium content (40% by weight) and its low cost.[70] It is sold under familiar trademark names such as Tums, Os-cal, and Caltrate. Other preparations with good bioavailability include calcium citrate, calcium lactate, and calcium citrate malate.[70] Bone meal dolomite and fossilized oyster shell preparations are not recommended due to the possibility of heavy metal contamination.[71]

Calcium citrate malate has been used in recent studies investigating the effect of calcium supplementation on bone acquisition in adolescents and children.[72,73] Calcium citrate malate has been shown to yield greater fractional absorption than calcium carbonate.[74] Calcium citrate malate is used commercially to fortify beverage products (Sunny Delight Plus Calcium; Hawaiian Punch Plus Calcium, Procter and Gamble, Cincinnati, Ohio).

Although studies demonstrate a positive effect of calcium supplementation on bone density,[72,73] the preferred method of achieving optimal calcium intake is through foods such as low-fat dairy products, broccoli, kale, calcium-set tofu, some legumes, canned fish, and nuts.

There is some concern that taking calcium supplements with meals will interfere with the absorption of other nutrients, particularly iron. Data show that calcium can inhibit iron absorption, particularly when these two nutrients are consumed together. Gleerup et al.[75] measured the absorption of iron from meals containing different amounts of dietary calcium and reported 30 to 50% more iron was absorbed when no milk or cheese was served. Cook et al.[76] observed that calcium supplements had little effect on iron absorption when taken without food. However, when consumed together, calcium reduced the absorption of iron by one third, particularly when taken with a test meal containing no meat, which is an important source of heme iron. According to Heaney,[77] iron interference should only be a problem for women with iron deficiency.

Excesses of one nutrient can create nutritional imbalances or increased requirements of other nutrients. Eating enough and a variety of foods are important ways of meeting total nutrient needs. Long-term studies are needed to further investigate the absorption, metabolism, and retention of calcium in humans in free-living situations.

III. IRON

Iron is present in all cells in the body. It helps transport oxygen, synthesize hemoglobin and myoglobin, and activate oxygen. Iron deficiency can affect several metabolic functions related to energy production. In addition to causing anemia, severe iron deficiency is known to decrease the capacity of skeletal muscle to consume oxygen and produce adenosine triphosphate, one of the major forms of energy available for immediate use in the body.[78]

Iron deserves special attention in sports nutrition because many female athletes do not consume enough and thus are at risk for iron deficiency. Iron deficiency is not only prevalent among female athletes but is also one of the most common nutritional deficiencies in the U.S. and the world. It occurs more often among women than men because of increased blood loss due to menstruation and inadequate dietary intake of iron as a result of low calorie intake. Exercise places additional demands on the body which may also affect iron status.

A. IRON ABSORPTION

Unlike other minerals, there is no physiological regulation of iron metabolism through increased or decreased excretion. The primary control for maintaining adequate levels of iron is the intestinal absorption system, which is influenced by an individual's iron status. Persons who are iron-deficient generally absorb a higher percentage of dietary iron than those who have sufficient iron.[79,80]

Several factors affect the absorption of iron including physiological demand for iron, dietary iron supply, and how efficiently the body uses the iron it has.[81] Whenever there is rapid growth, such as during adolescence or pregnancy, the need for iron increases. According to Hallberg and Rossander-Hulten,[82] adolescent girls require an additional 0.38 mg/d of iron to cover the requirements for growth. The iron requirement for pregnant women is between 420 to 1030 mg/d or approximately 1 to 2.5 mg/d over the 15 months of pregnancy and lactation.[83]

Although an individual's iron stores are the principal determinant of iron absorption, bioavailability of iron is also an important factor. Iron is absorbed as heme and nonheme, and its availability from food sources varies greatly. Heme iron (meat, poultry, fish) is well absorbed (15 to 35%) by the body, regardless of the composition of a meal.[84] Nonheme iron, found primarily in plant foods, is not well absorbed (2 to 20%). The rate of nonheme absorption depends on enhancing and inhibiting substances in the diet.[85] Meat, fish, poultry, and ascorbic acid increase nonheme iron availability,[86] while tea, coffee, calcium, and bran inhibit iron absorption.[81] Morck et al.[87] reported that a glass of tea reduced iron absorption from a hamburger meal by 64%.

B. IRON STATUS OF FEMALE ATHLETES

Several investigators have examined the iron status of female athletes.[89-95] In a study comprising 100 female athletes and 66 nonathletes, Risser et al.[95] reported that 31% of the athletes and 45% of the nonathletes were iron deficient as determined by serum ferritin (<12 µg/l) and transferrin saturation levels (<16%). Iron deficiency without anemia was more common than anemia; only 7% of the athletes had hemoglobin levels of <12 g/l. In another study, Balaban et al.[88] concluded that iron deficiency in athletes is no more frequent than in the general population, about 25%. However, the incidence of iron deficiency is reportedly greater in female than in male athletes,[89,92] and athletes consuming vegetarian diets.[96,97]

C. MEASURES OF IRON STATUS

A deficiency of iron develops gradually, progressing through several stages before anemia is evident.[98] Iron depletion is the first stage, as reflected by a decrease in serum ferritin concentration. According to Harris et al.,[99] normal serum ferritin levels for female athletes range from 30 to 150 µg/l, with 30 µg/ml being an average value. A serum ferritin level of less than 20 µg/l represents minimal iron stores, and a value of less than 12 µg/l represents complete depletion of iron stores in the bone marrow.[99] Some researchers classify athletes as iron-depleted based on serum ferritin measurements alone, where other researchers use several parameters.

The second stage of iron deficiency is marked by a fall in transferrin saturation levels (<16%) and an increase in free erythrocyte protoporphyrin (>100 µg/dl), indicating the production of red blood cells with insufficient iron. In the third stage, iron deficiency anemia is evidenced by a significant decline in circulating hemoglobin (<12 g/l in women), a decrease in mean corpuscular volume, and hypochromic, microcytic blood cells indicating red blood cells are abnormally small due to poor hemoglobinization. Low hemoglobin levels do not always mean anemia or the need for iron supplementation. To determine if a borderline hemoglobin level in an athlete is indicative of anemia, the value should be compared to the athlete's baseline level.[99]

Female athletes should be screened once a year to detect early stages of iron depletion. A comprehensive evaluation should include a complete blood count, information on diet, weight control behaviors, drug usage (i.e., aspirin, inflammatory agents), and menstrual history. Laboratory tests of iron status are subject to variation during the phases of the menstrual cycle. In a study by Kim et al.,[100] mean values of hemoglobin, transferrin saturation, and serum ferritin were lowest during menses and highest in the luteal or late luteal phase. Thus surveys examining the iron status of female athletes should control for the different phases of the menstrual cycle.

D. CAUSES OF IRON DEFICIENCY

A number of factors can contribute to iron deficiency in female athletes, including heavy training,[101] gastrointestinal bleeding,[92,102] red blood cell hemolysis,[103] increased iron losses through sweating,[104] decreased iron absorption,[96,97] and inadequate dietary intake.

In endurance athletes, the cause of low serum iron levels may be related to what Dickson et al.[101] refers to as "dilutional anemia" or hemodilution. Prolonged exercise expands plasma volume, diluting the red blood cells and thus temporarily lowering hemoglobin levels. In many cases, hemoglobin levels return to normal when training is reduced.

Another possible contributing factor to decreased iron levels in some athletes is gastrointestinal blood loss. Nickerson et al.[92] studied female cross-country runners and reported that 34% had decreased iron stores with serum ferritin levels below 12 μg/l. The main reasons found for iron deficiency in this study were low initial iron stores and gastrointestinal bleeding, which occurred in 9 out of 20 female runners. In a study that compared bowel function, fecal hemoglobin loss and iron status of female runners, Lampe et al.[102] reported that 5 out of 35 women had gastrointestinal bleeding during the study period. Thus, some women may be more prone to gastrointestinal bleeding than others.

The female athlete faces a potentially greater loss of iron as a result of menstruation. The average monthly menstrual blood loss is between 20 and 30 ml.[105] Oral contraceptives significantly reduce iron losses while increased losses have been observed with intrauterine devices.[105]

As previously mentioned, the amount of iron absorbed in the body depends on the individual's iron status, the form of iron, and the presence of enhancers and inhibitors. Heme iron in animal foods is absorbed and utilized more readily than nonheme iron in plant foods (fruits, vegetables, grains, and cereals). Meat has a two-fold effect on iron absorption; it is an excellent source of bioavailable heme iron, and it promotes the absorption of nonheme iron.[105] The presence of vitamin C also increases nonheme iron absorption, although recent evidence suggests that it may have a more modest effect on iron absorption than previously thought.[106]

Female athletes consuming vegetarian diets may be at risk for iron deficiency due to poor absorption of nonheme iron. Snyder et al.[96] reported the bioavailability of iron was significantly lower in female runners consuming a modified vegetarian diet (less than 100 g red meat/week), than in runners consuming red meat, 0.66 mg/d vs. 0.91 mg/d, respectively. No differences were noted in total calorie intake and both groups consumed approximately 14 mg/d of dietary iron. The athletes who ate red meat consumed more heme iron (1.2 mg/d) than the athletes consuming a modified vegetarian diet (0.2 mg/d). Fetherman et al.[107] reported similar results in another study involving female runners. The mean iron intake of the subjects met the RDA of 15 mg/d, but the mean bioavailability of iron was low at 1.06 mg/d, suggesting that nonheme sources of iron were more prevalent in the diet.

Based on calculations by Hallberg and Rossander-Hulten,[82] the amount of iron needed to be absorbed to cover the iron requirements of menstruating women is 2.84 mg/d. To assure this amount, the diet should provide 18.9 mg/d of available iron (heme and nonheme) or approximately 9.4 mg/1000 kcal/d for a female consuming approximately 2000 kcal/d. Manore et al.[108] reported that a group of female runners averaged 6 mg iron/1000 kcal with a range of 4.3 to 8.8 mg iron/1000 kcal. The runners consumed less than 85 g (3 oz.) of meat, fish, or poultry a day; only 11 to 14% of dietary iron was from animal sources (4 to 6% heme iron).

In addition to decreased iron absorption, inadequate dietary iron intake is a major contributing factor to the prevalence of iron deficiency in female athletes.[109,110] The RDA for iron is 15 mg/d for women.[111] Many groups of female athletes, particularly young gymnasts, consume less than the RDA for iron. Reggiani et al.[112] evaluated the diets of 26 adolescent gymnasts and reported a mean iron intake of 6.2 mg/d with a range of 2.7 to 12.6. In another study involving 26 female college gymnasts and a control group, mean dietary iron intakes were 11.8 mg/d and 12.4 mg/d, respectively.[113] Low mean iron intakes were also noted in gymnasts studied by Moffatt,[114] Loosli et al.,[115] and Benardot et al.[116]

Low energy intakes and decreased consumption of red meat are two primary reasons why females' diets are low in iron. Data from the third National Health and Nutrition Examination Survey (NHANES III) reported that females 16 to 19 years old averaged 1,274 kcal/d and 12.5 mg/d of iron.[117,118] Dietary surveys of female adolescent athletes show mean energy intakes ranging from 1706 to 3572 kcal/d, with an average of 13 mg/d of iron (Table 1.4). Many dancers,[119,120] and gymnasts[112,113,116] consume less than 1800 kcal/d, and as a result, limit their intake of dietary iron.

However, even in adolescents consuming meat, nutritional deficiencies of iron and poor iron status can result from low calorie intakes. Donovan and Gibson[121] assessed the iron and zinc status of 124 young females, aged 14 to 19 years, consuming vegetarian, semi-vegetarian, and omnivorous diets. Results showed that mean energy intakes were below recommended levels for all three groups. Intakes of meat, poultry, and fish were low even in the omnivorous group, resulting in a correspondingly lower contribution of heme iron to total dietary iron intake.

Athletes should include at least 85 g (3 oz) of meat, fish, or poultry a day and consume a good source of vitamin C. The food composition information in Table 4.5 shows the difference between total iron content and the amount of available iron from heme and nonheme food sources.

TABLE 4.5   Total Iron Content and Amount of Available Iron From Heme and Nonheme Food Sources

Food (3 oz. cooked, lean only)		Total Iron (mg)	Available Iron (mg)	Food		Total Iron (mg)	Available Iron (mg)
Beef	Liver, pan fried	5.34	0.60	Grains	Bagel, 1	1.80	0.09
	Chuck, arm pot roast, braised	3.22	0.48		Bran muffin, home recipe, 1	1.40	0.07
	Tenderloin, roasted	3.05	0.46		Whole wheat bread, 1 sl.	1.00	0.05
	Sirloin, broiled	2.85	0.42		White rice (enriched), cooked, 1/2 c	0.90	0.05
	Roundtip, roasted	2.50	0.38		White bread (enriched), 1 sl.	0.70	0.04
	Top round, broiled	2.10	0.31		Brown rice, cooked, 1/2 c	0.50	0.03
	Ground lean, broiled	1.79	0.27	Fruits	Apricots, dried, 7 halves	1.16	0.06
	Eye round, roasted	1.65	0.25		Prunes, dried, 3 med.	0.84	0.04
Pork	Shoulder, blade, Boston, roasted	1.36	0.15		Raisins, 2 Tbsp.	0.38	0.02
	Tenderloin, roasted	1.31	0.15		Banana, 1 med.	0.35	0.02
	Ham boneless, 5–11% fat	1.19	0.14		Apple, 1 med.	0.25	0.01
	Loin chop broiled	0.78	0.09		Orange, 1 med.	0.13	0.01
Lamb	Loin, roasted	2.07	0.31	Vegetables	Potato, baked w/skin, 1 med.	2.75	0.14
	Leg, shank half, roasted	1.75	0.26		Peas, cooked, 1/2 c	1.26	0.06
Veal	Loin, roasted	0.93	0.14		Spinach, raw, 1/2 c	0.76	0.04
	Cutlet, pan fried	0.74	0.11		Broccoli, raw, 1/2 c	0.39	0.02

Chicken	Liver, simmered	7.20	0.81
	Leg, roasted	1.11	0.17
	Breast, roasted	0.88	0.13
Turkey	Leg, roasted	2.26	0.34
	Breast, roasted	0.99	0.14
Fish	Tuna, light meat, canned	2.72	0.31
	white meat, canned	0.51	0.06
	Halibut, dry heat	0.91	0.10
	Salmon, sockeye, dry heat	0.47	0.06
	Flounder/sole, dry heat	0.23	0.03
Shellfish	Oysters, 6 medium, raw	5.63	0.63
	Shrimp, moist heat	2.63	0.30
	Crab, Alaskan king, moist heat	0.65	0.07
Cereals	Raisin bran (enrich), dry, 1/2 c	4.50	0.23
	Corn flakes (enrich), dry, 1 oz	1.80	0.09
	Shredded wheat, dry, 1 oz	1.20	0.06
	Oatmeal, cooked, 1/2 c	0.80	0.04
	Whole wheat hot cereal, 1/2 c	0.75	0.04
Beans/Legumes	Carrots, 1 med.	0.36	0.02
	Lettuce, iceberg, 1/8 head	0.34	0.02
	Corn, cooked, 1/2 c	0.25	0.01
	Kidney beans, boiled, 1/2 c	2.58	0.13
	canned, 1/2 c	1.57	0.08
	Chickpeas, boiled, 1/2 c	2.37	0.12
	canned, 1/2 c	1.62	0.08
	Baked beans, canned, plain, 1/2 c	0.37	0.02
Meat Substitutes	Tofu, 1 1/2 × 2 3/4 × 1 in.	2.30	0.12
	Egg, whole	1.00	0.05
	yolk	0.95	0.05
	white	tr	—
	Peanut butter, 2 Tbsp	0.60	0.03
Dairy	Milk, lowfat, 1 c	0.12	0.01
	Yogurt, plain lowfat, 1 c	0.18	0.01
	Cheese, cheddar, 1 oz	0.19	0.01
Molasses	Cane, blackstrap, 1 Tbsp	5.05	0.25

From *Iron in Human Nutrition*, National Live Stock and Meat Board, 1990. With permission.

E. EFFECTS OF IRON DEFICIENCY ON PERFORMANCE

It is well known that iron deficiency anemia can compromise athletic performance,[78] but the effects of nonanemic iron deficiency are less clear. One way in which investigators have addressed this issue is by examining the effects of iron supplementation on performance in iron-deficient athletes. Klingshirn et al.[122] studied the effects of iron supplementation (160 mg/d of ferrous sulfate) on endurance performance in initially iron-depleted nonanemic (serum ferritin <20 µg/l; hemoglobin >12 g/dl) female distance runners. Eight weeks of iron supplementation resulted in a rise in mean serum ferritin levels from 11.6 µg/l to 23.4 µg/l, while hemoglobin levels remained constant. Subjects performed a VO_{2max} test and endurance run to exhaustion. There were no significant differences between the experimental and control groups with respect to physical performance. Similar results were reported by Fogelholm et al.[123]

In another study, Newhouse et al.[109] reported that 8 weeks of iron supplementation (320 mg/d ferrous sulfate) administered to iron deficient female runners did not enhance work capacity. Serum ferritin values increased from 12.4 µg/l to 37.7 µg/l for the experimental group and from 12.2 µg/l to 17.2 µg/d for the control group. In contrast, Rowland et al.[124] reported that iron-deficient female runners receiving ferrous sulfate (975 mg/d) for 4 weeks increased treadmill endurance times compared to a control group.

According to Telford et al.,[125] nonanemic athletes with a serum ferritin level of 20 µg/l should not be concerned about their ability to perform an endurance event. However, it would seem prudent for female athletes with serum ferritin levels less than 20 µg/l to increase their iron stores through the diet or take a multivitamin providing 100% of the RDA for iron, to avoid risk of developing iron deficiency.

One area currently being investigated is the relationship between low iron stores and overuse injuries in female athletes. Similar to the theory that inadequate dietary calcium may contribute to low bone mineral density and risk for osteoporosis, Loosli et al.[126] have hypothesized that inadequate dietary iron may contribute to reduced iron stores and risk for injury. In a preliminary study of 101 female cross-country runners, Loosli et al.[126] found that athletes with the lowest serum ferritin levels (<13.7 µg/ml) had twice as many overuse injuries as athletes with normal serum ferritin levels (>24 µg/ml). Athletes with the lowest serum ferritins had lower mean iron intakes (10.2 mg/d) and consumed fewer calories (1,632 kcal/d) than the athletes with normal ferritin levels, 15.3 mg/d and 1,964 kcal/d, respectively. According to Loosli et al.,[126] low iron stores may predispose muscles and tendons to fatigue or slow ongoing muscle and tendon repair.

Although the strongest predictors of overuse injuries in runners are history of previous injury, weekly mileage, and running experience,[127] nutritional deficiencies play a role. An athlete with a poor diet risks poor health, illness, and injury, all of which affect the ability to train and compete.

F. IRON SUPPLEMENTATION

Iron supplementation is prevalent among athletes, particularly female runners.[66,68,69,128-131] In a study of 103 women runners, Pate et al.[68] reported that 50% took iron supplements. Deuster et al.[66] found that 59% of regular menstruating runners and 41% of amenorrheic runners took supplements. Iron was the supplement most frequently used and some athletes reported consuming more than 50 mg/d.

Athletes who are iron deficient should receive diet counseling and, when indicated, supplemental iron; 300 mg/d of ferrous sulfate is commonly prescribed. The athlete should be informed about the types and sources of dietary iron to augment treatment.

Recent studies have shown that supplementation on a weekly basis or two to three times per week with a relatively low dose of iron is as effective as daily administration in improving iron status of persons with low iron stores.[132-134] The basis for giving iron supplements weekly is that cumulative daily doses of iron rapidly reduce the intestinal absorption of iron.[135] It is also believed that compliance is improved by decreasing the negative side effects which often accompany use of iron supplements. However, Cook and Reddy[136] found no advantage in giving iron less than once daily to healthy young women with marginal iron stores.

One concern with taking iron supplements is the interaction with other nutrients. Studies have reported decreased absorption of zinc and copper with iron supplements.[137-139] In susceptible individuals, long-term iron supplementation can also lead to toxicity or iron overload, which is a serious complication caused by abnormal absorption of iron in the body. There are two kinds of iron overload. One is caused by prolonged administration of iron to individuals who are not iron deficient. The other is caused by hereditary hemochromatosis, an inborn error of metabolism in which increased intestinal absorption of iron results in a slow progressive accumulation of iron throughout life.[83] It is estimated that two to three out of every 1000 people in the U.S. are homozygous for the iron-overloading gene. Therefore, the risk for iron overload, although more prevalent in men than women, deserves attention.

IV. ZINC

A. FUNCTIONS OF ZINC

Zinc is an essential trace mineral found in minute amounts in all organs, tissues, fluids, and secretions of the body.[140] It is a component of many enzymes involved in the metabolism of protein, carbohydrates, and fat. Zinc also influences the activity of several hormones such as growth hormone, thyroid hormone, and sex hormones. Optimal zinc is needed for growth and for proper immune function. An adequate zinc status helps the body fight off infections caused by viruses and bacteria.[140]

The RDA for zinc is 12 mg/d for females.[141] This is based on an assumed average requirement of 2.5 mg/d of absorbed zinc. The requirement for zinc is greatest during periods of rapid growth, such as adolescence and pregnancy.

B. FOOD SOURCES OF ZINC

Zinc is widely distributed in animal and plant foods. Meat, liver, oysters, eggs, seafood, and legumes are the most nutrient-dense sources of zinc (Table 4.6). Milk and milk products are also important sources of zinc. Mares-Perlman et al.[142] reported that in women over 65 years of age milk was the most prevalent source of zinc, accounting for 18.5% and 21.9% of dietary zinc, respectively. Some foods, such as white bread, coffee, and tea can contribute greatly to zinc intake because they are frequently consumed.[142] Additionally, many fortified ready-to-eat cereals contain up to 25% of the Daily Value for zinc.

Like iron, the important issue in the diet is the total amount of zinc absorbed from food. This is influenced in part by an individual's zinc status. Zinc absorption increases when zinc intakes are low and decreases when zinc intakes are high.[140] Foods from animal sources (meat, liver, eggs, and seafood) increase zinc bioavailability, while phytates and fiber can greatly inhibit zinc absorption.[143,144]

C. ZINC STATUS OF FEMALE ATHLETES

Studies have shown that compared to nonathletes, female athletes have lower than normal serum zinc levels (<11.5 µmol/l).[145-147] Haralambie[147] measured serum zinc concentrations in 160 athletes (57 women and 103 men) and found that 43% of the women had suboptimal zinc levels. In another study by Deuster et al.,[66] 12 of 51 female runners had serum zinc levels <12 µmol/l. Whether suboptimal zinc status impairs athletic performance is not known.

Several factors have been associated with decreased serum zinc levels in female athletes including lower dietary intake and/or absorption of zinc,[145,146] increased zinc losses in sweat,[148] and increased zinc losses in urine.[145] Additionally, training intensity may alter zinc status. Couzy et al.[149] found a significant decrease in serum zinc after 5 months of increased training in male runners, despite an adequate intake of dietary zinc. More recent data suggests, however, that serum may not be an appropriate measure for evaluating zinc stores. Dolev et al.[150] examined zinc content in serum, red blood cells, and mononuclear cells (MNCs) in 23 male military recruits during a 12-week progressive exercise program. Zinc content in mononuclear cells increased during strenuous training, but no changes in serum zinc or red blood cells were noted. Further research is needed to determine a more reliable indicator of zinc status.

Females are more likely to consume inadequate intakes of zinc because of lower energy intakes and/or lower intakes of meat.[121,142] Nowak et al.[151] compared the nutrient intake of male and female basketball players and

TABLE 4.6

Food Sources of Zinc ✿

RDA for women: 12 mg/d

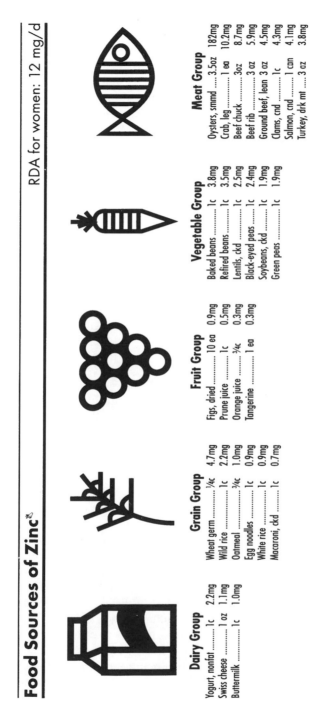

Dairy Group

Yogurt, nonfat	1c	2.2mg
Swiss cheese	1 oz	1.1mg
Buttermilk	1c	1.0mg

Grain Group

Wheat germ	¼c	4.7mg
Wild rice	1c	2.2mg
Oatmeal	¾c	1.0mg
Egg noodles	1c	0.9mg
White rice	1c	0.9mg
Macaroni, ckd	1c	0.7mg

Fruit Group

Figs, dried	10 ea	0.9mg
Prune juice	1c	0.5mg
Orange juice	¾c	0.3mg
Tangerine	1 ea	0.3mg

Vegetable Group

Baked beans	1c	3.8mg
Refried beans	1c	3.5mg
Lentils, ckd	1c	2.5mg
Black-eyed peas	1c	2.4mg
Soybeans, ckd	1c	1.9mg
Green peas	1c	1.9mg

Meat Group

Oysters, smmd	3.5oz	182mg
Crab, leg	1 ea	10.2mg
Beef chuck	3oz	8.7mg
Beef rib	3 oz	5.9mg
Ground beef, lean	3 oz	4.5mg
Clams, cnd	1c	4.3mg
Salmon, cnd	1 can	4.1mg
Turkey, drk mt	3 oz	3.8mg

✿ An excellent source provides more than 3.0 mg per serving

reported a significantly lower mean zinc intake among the female athletes (7 ± 3 mg/d) than the male athletes (17 ± 6 mg/d), which the authors attributed to the women's low mean energy intake (1,730 ± 573 kcal/d) and dietary patterns. Both of these factors may limit the amount of zinc absorbed from food and thereby compromise zinc nutritional status. In another study, Singh et al.[146] found that despite adequate intakes of dietary zinc, female runners had lower serum zinc concentrations. The authors believed this may have been due to decreased zinc absorption. The runner's diets were reportedly high in dietary fiber, which binds zinc and makes it less available to the body.

D. ZINC SUPPLEMENTATION

As female athletes learn more about the role of zinc in health and performance, the use of zinc supplements may become more prevalent. In a study of supplementation patterns in marathon runners, Nieman et al.[128] found that 29% of runners reported daily use of at least one type of supplement. Approximately 4% of the total group took zinc supplements. Of that 4%, 7.5% were over the age of 45.

There are some adverse consequences to consuming high levels of zinc over a long period of time. Zinc can interfere with the metabolism of other nutrients, particularly copper and iron.[140] Excess amounts of zinc can cause nausea, vomiting, abdominal pain, fatigue, and anemia.

V. CONCLUSIONS

Several studies have reported inadequate dietary intakes of calcium, iron, and zinc among female athletes. These three minerals perform specific functions in the body and thereby play important roles in health and performance. Inadequate dietary calcium can contribute to low bone density and risk for osteoporosis. Athletes who do not consume enough dietary iron risk iron depletion and impaired performance. Generally when dietary iron intake is low, so is zinc because food sources (meat, fish, poultry) of these two minerals are similar.

The body's ability to absorb and utilize calcium, iron, and zinc is greatly affected by the presence of other nutrients and dietary substances as well as physiological factors. Factors which increase calcium absorption include vitamin D, estrogen, and exercise. Meat increases the absorption of iron and zinc.

While many factors can contribute to a deficiency, inadequate dietary intake is the most likely cause. Female athletes who are dieting or consuming vegetarian diets should be encouraged to include low-fat dairy products and lean meats in the diet. Those who do not consume significant amounts of these minerals will benefit from a multivitamin/mineral providing no more than 100% of the RDA. A concern with taking supplements is the interaction with other nutrients.

REFERENCES

1. Barger-Lux, M. J. and Heaney, R. P., The role of calcium intake in preventing bone fragility, hypertension, and certain cancers, *J. Nutr.*, 124, 1406S, 1994.
2. Food and Nutrition Board, National Research Council, *Recommended Dietary Allowances*, 10th ed., National Academy Press, Washington, D.C., 1989, 179.
3. Fleming, K. H. and Heimbach, J. T., Consumption of calcium in the U.S.: Food sources and intake levels, *J. Nutr.*, 124, 1426S, 1994.
4. Chapman, K. M., Chan, M. W., and Clark, C. D., Factors influencing dairy calcium intake in women, *J. Am. Coll. Nutr.*, 14, 336, 1995.
5. Grandjean, A. C., unpublished data, 1991.
6. Webster, B. L. and Barr, S. I., Calcium intakes of adolescent female gymnasts and speed skaters: lack of association with dieting behavior, *Int. J. Sport Nutr.*, 5, 2, 1995.
7. Karanja, N., Morris, C. D., Rufolo, P., Snyder, G., Illingworth, D. R., and McCarron, D. A., Impact of increasing calcium in the diet on nutrient consumption, plasma lipids, and lipoproteins in humans, *Am. J. Clin. Nutr.*, 59, 900, 1994.
8. Weaver, C. M. and Plawecki, K. L., Dietary calcium: adequacy of a vegetarian diet, *Am. J. Clin. Nutr.*, 59, 1238S, 1994.
9. Optimal Calcium Intake. NIH Consensus Statement, June 6-8; 12, 1, 1994.
10. Porter, D. V., Washington update: NIH consensus development conference statement optimal calcium intake, *Nutr. Today*, 29, 37, September/October, 1994.
11. Matkovic, V., Fontana, D., Tominac, C., Goel, P., and Chestnut III, C. H., Factors that influence peak bone mass formation: a study of calcium balance and the inheritance of bone mass in adolescent females, *Am. J. Clin. Nutr.*, 52, 878, 1990.
12. Abrams, S. A. and Stuff, J. E., Calcium metabolism in girls: current dietary intakes lead to low rates of calcium absorption and retention during puberty, *Am. J. Clin. Nutr.*, 60, 739, 1994.
13. Lee, W. T. K., Leung, S. S. F., Wang, S., Xu, Y., Zeng, W., Lau, J., Oppenheimer, S. J., and Cheng, J. C. Y., Double-blind, controlled calcium supplementation and bone mineral accretion in children accustomed to a low-calcium diet, *Am. J. Clin. Nutr.*, 60, 744, 1994.
14. Andon, M. B., Lloyd, T., and Matkovic, V., Supplementation trials with calcium citrate malate: evidence in favor of increasing the calcium RDA during childhood and adolescence, *J. Nutr.*, 124, 1412S, 1994.
15. Matkovic, V. and Heaney, R. P., Calcium balance during human growth: evidence for threshold behavior, *Am. J. Clin. Nutr.*, 55, 992, 1992.
16. Matkovic, V., Ilich, J. Z., Andon, M. B., Hsieh, L. C., Tzagournis, M. A., Lagger, B. J., and Goel, P. K., Urinary calcium, sodium, and bone mass of young females, *Am. J. Clin. Nutr.*, 62, 417, 1995.
17. Halioua, L. and Anderson, J. J. B., Lifetime calcium intake and physical activity habits: independent and combined effects on the radial bone of healthy premenopausal Caucasian women, *Am. J. Clin. Nutr.*, 49, 534, 1989.
18. Baran, D., Sorensen, A., Grimes, J., Lew, R., Karellas, A., Johnson, B., and Roche, J., Dietary modification with dairy products for preventing vertebral bone loss in premenopausal women: a three-year prospective study, *J. Clin. Endocrinol. Metab.*, 70, 264, 1990.
19. Hu, J., Zhao, X., Jia, J., Parpia, B., and Campbell, T. C., Dietary calcium and bone density among middle-aged and elderly women in China, *Am. J. Clin. Nutr.*, 58, 219, 1993.
20. Chapuy, M. C., Arlot, M. E., Duboeuf, F., Brun, J., Crouzet, B., Arnaud, S., Delmas, P. D., and Meunier, P. J., Vitamin D_3 and calcium to prevent hip fractures in elderly women, *N. Engl. J. Med.*, 327, 1637, 1992.
21. Reid, I. R., Ames, R. W., Evans, M. C., Gamble, G. D., and Sharpe, S. J., Long-term effects of calcium supplementation on bone loss and fractures in postmenopausal women: a randomized controlled trial, *Amer. J. Med.*, 98, 331, 1995.

22. Weaver, C. M., Martin, B. R., Plawecki, K. L., Peacock, M., Wood, O. B., Smith, D. L., and Wastney, M. E., Differences in calcium metabolism between adolescent and adult females, *Am. J. Clin. Nutr.*, 61, 577, 1995.
23. Heaney, R. P., Protein intake and the calcium economy, *J. Am. Diet. Assoc.*, 93, 1259, 1993.
24. Metz, J. A., Anderson, J. J. B., and Gallagher, P. N., Jr., Intakes of calcium, phosphorus, and protein, and physical-activity level are related to radial bone mass in young adult women, *Am. J. Clin. Nutr.*, 58, 537, 1993.
25. Heaney, R. P. and Recker, R. R., Effects of nitrogen, phosphorus, and caffeine on calcium balance in women, *J. Lab. Clin. Med.*, 99, 46, 1982.
26. Wardlaw, G. M., Putting osteoporosis in perspective, *J. Am. Diet. Assoc.*, 93, 1000, 1993.
27. Harris, S. S. and Dawson-Hughes, B., Caffeine and bone loss in healthy postmenopausal women, *Am. J. Clin. Nutr.*, 60, 573, 1994.
28. Lloyd, T., Schaeffer, J. M., Walker, M. A., and Demers, L. M., Urinary hormonal concentrations and spinal bone densities of premenopausal vegetarian and nonvegetarian women, *Am. J. Clin. Nutr.*, 54, 1005, 1991.
29. Heaney, R. P., Weaver, C. M., and Fitzsimmons, M. L., Soybean phytate content: effect on calcium absorption, *Am. J. Clin. Nutr.*, 53, 745, 1991.
30. Heaney, R. P., Weaver, C. M., and Recker, R. R., Calcium absorbability from spinach, *Am. J. Clin. Nutr.*, 47, 707, 1988.
31. Heaney, R. P. and Weaver, C. M., Calcium absorption from kale, *Am. J. Clin. Nutr.*, 51, 656, 1990.
32. Weaver, C. M., Heaney, R. P., Martin, B. R., and Fitzsimmons, M. L., Human calcium absorption from whole-wheat products, *J. Nutr.*, 121, 1769, 1991.
33. Conference Report, Consensus development conference: prophylaxis and treatment of osteoporosis, *Am. J. Med.*, 90, 107, 1991.
34. Melton III, L. J., How many women have osteoporosis now?, *J. Bone Mineral Res.*, 10, 175, 1995.
35. Delmas, P. D., Introduction, *Am. J. Med.*, 98 (Suppl 2A), 2A-1S, 1995.
36. Lindsay, R. The burden of osteoporosis: cost, *Am. J. Med.*, (Suppl 2A), 2A-9S, 1995.
37. Heaney, R. P., Saville, P. D., and Recker, R. R., Calcium absorption as a function of calcium intake, *J. Lab. Clin. Med.*, 85, 881, 1975.
38. Heaney, R. P., Gallagher, T. C., Johnson, C. C., Neer, R., Parfitt, A. M., and Whedon, G. D., Calcium nutrition and bone health in the elderly, *Am. J. Clin. Nutr.*, 36, 986, 1982.
39. Richelson, L. S., Wahner, H. W., Melton, L. J., and Riggs, B. L., Relative contributions of aging and estrogen deficiency to postmenopausal bone loss, *N. Engl. J. Med.*, 311, 1273, 1984.
40. Heaney, R. P., Nutritional factors and estrogen in age-related bone loss, *Clin. Invest. Med.*, 5, 147, 1982.
41. Aloia, J. F., Cohn, S. H., Ostuni, J. A., Cane, R., and Ellis, K., Prevention of involutional bone loss by exercise, *Ann. Int. Med.*, 89, 356, 1978.
42. Anderson, J. J. B. and Metz, J. A., Contributions of dietary calcium and physical activity to primary prevention of osteoporosis in females, *J. Am. Coll. Nutr.*, 12, 378, 1993.
43. Suominen, H., Bone mineral density and long term exercise, *Sports Med.*, 16, 316, 1993.
44. Nilsson, B. E. and Westlin, N. E., Bone density in athletes, *Clin. Orthop. Rel. Res.*, 77, 179, 1971.
45. Heinrich, C. H., Going, S. B., Pamenter, R. W., Perry, C. D., Boyden, T. W., and Lohman, T. G., Bone mineral content of cyclically menstruating female resistance and endurance trained athletes, *Med. Sci. Sports Exerc.*, 22, 558, 1990.
46. Yeager, K. K., Agostini, R., Nattiv, A., and Drinkwater, B., The female athlete triad: disordered eating, amenorrhea, osteoporosis, *Med. Sci. Sports Exerc.*, 25, 775, 1993.
47. Nelson, M. E., Fisher, E. C., Catsos, P. D., Meredith, C. N., Turksoy, R. N., and Evans, W. J., Diet and bone status in amenorrheic runners, *Am. J. Clin. Nutr.*, 43, 910, 1986.

48. Emans, S. J., Grace, E., Hoffer, F. A., Gundberg, C., Ravnikar, V., and Woods, E. R., Estrogen deficiency in adolescents and young adults: Impact on bone mineral content and effects of estrogen replacement therapy, *Obstet. Gynecol.*, 76, 585, 1990.

49. Micklesfield, L. K., Lambert, E. V., Fataar, A. B., Noakes, T. D., and Myburgh, K. H., Bone mineral density in mature, premenopausal ultramarathon runners, *Med. Sci. Sports Exerc.*, 688, 1995.

50. Putukian, M., The female triad. Eating disorders, amenorrhea, and osteoporosis, *Med. Clin. North Amer.*, 78, 345, 1994.

51. Schweiger, U., Laessle, R., Schweiger, M., Herrmann, F., Riedel, W., and Pirke, K., Calorie intake, stress, and menstrual function in athletes, *Fertil. Steril.*, 49, 447, 1988.

52. Wolman, R. L. and Harries, M. G., Menstrual abnormalities in elite athletes, *Clin. Sports Med.*, 1, 95, 1989.

53. Kaiserauer S., Snyder, A. C., Sleeper, M., and Zierath, J., Nutritional, physiological, and menstrual status of distance runners, *Med. Sci. Sports Exerc.*, 21, 120, 1989.

54. Baer, J. T. and Taper, L. J., Amenorrheic and eumenorrheic adolescent runners: dietary intake and exercise training status, *J. Am. Diet. Assoc.*, 91, 89, 1992.

55. Marcus, R., Cann, C., Madvig, P., Minkoff, J., Goddard, M., Bayer, M., Martin, M., Gaudiani, L., Haskell, W. and Genant, H., Menstrual function and bone mass in elite women distance runners, *Ann. Int. Med.*, 102, 158, 1985.

56. Fisher, E. C., Nelson, M. E., Frontera, W. R., Turksoy, R. N., and Evans, W. J., Bone mineral content and levels of gonadotropins and estrogens in amenorrheic running women, *J. Clin. Endocrinol. Metab.*, 62, 1232, 1986.

57. Benson, J. E., Geiger, C. J., Eiserman, P. A., and Wardlaw, G. M., Relationship between nutrient intake, body mass index, menstrual function, and ballet injury, *J. Am. Diet. Assoc.*, 89, 58, 1989.

58. Myburgh, K. H., Bachrach, L. K., Lewis, B., Kent, K., and Marcus, R., Low bone mineral density at axial and appendicular sites in amenorrheic athletes, *Med. Sci. Sports Exerc.*, 25, 1197, 1993.

59. Drinkwater, B. L., Nilson, K., Chestnut, C. H. III, Bremner, W. J., Shainholtz, S., and Southworth, M. B., Bone mineral content of amenorrheic and eumenorrheic athletes, *N. Engl. J. Med.*, 311, 277, 1984.

60. Warren, M. P., Brooks-Gunn, J., Hamilton, L. H., Warren, L. F., and Hamilton, W. G., Scoliosis and fractures in young ballet dancers, *N. Engl. J. Med.*, 314, 1348, 1986.

61. Sutton, J. R. and Nilson, K. L., Repeated stress fractures in an amenorrheic marathoner, *Phys. Sportsmed.*, 17, 65, 1989.

62. Frusztajer, N. T., Dhuper, S., Warren, M. P., Brooks-Gunn, J., and Fox, R. P., Nutrition and the incidence of stress fractures in ballet dancers, *Am. J. Clin. Nutr.*, 51, 779, 1990.

63. Drinkwater, B. L., Bruemner, B., and Chesnut, C. H., Menstrual history as a determinant of current bone density in young athletes, *J. Am. Med. Assoc.*, 263, 545, 1990.

64. Jonnavithula, S., Warren, M. P., Fox, R. P., and Lazaro, M. I., Bone density is compromised in amenorrheic women despite return of menses: a 2-year study, *Obstet. Gynecol.*, 81, 669, 1993.

65. Constantini, N. W., Clinical consequences of athletic amenorrhoea, *Sports Med.*, 17, 213, 1994.

66. Deuster, P. A., Kyle, S. B., Moser, P. B., Vigersky, R. A., Singh, A., and Schoomaker, E. B., Nutritional survey of highly trained women runners, *Am. J. Clin. Nutr.*, 44, 954, 1986.

67. Sobal, J. and Marquart, L. F., Vitamin/mineral supplement use among athletes: a review of the literature, *Int. J. Sport Nutr.*, 4, 320, 1994.

68. Pate, R. R., Sargent, R. G., Baldwin, C., and Burgess, M. L., Dietary intake of women runners, *Int. J. Sports Med.*, 11, 461, 1990.

69. Barr, S. I., Nutrition knowledge and selected nutritional practices of female recreational athletes, *J. Nutr. Educ.*, 18, 167, 1986.

70. Levenson, D. I. and Bockman, R. S., A review of calcium preparations, *Nutr. Rev.*, 52, 221, 1994.

71. Whiting, S. J., Safety of some calcium supplements questioned, *Nutr. Rev.*, 52, 95, 1994.

72. Johnston, C. C., Miller, J. Z., Slemenda, C. W., Reister, T. K., Hui, S., Christian, J. C., and Peacock, M., Calcium supplementation and increases in bone mineral density in children, *N. Engl. J. Med.*, 327, 82, 1992.

73. Lloyd, T., Andon, M. B., Rollings, N., Martel, J. K., Landis, J. R., Demers, L. M., Eggli, D. F., Kieselhorst, K., and Kulin, H. E., Calcium supplementation and bone mineral density in adolescent girls, *J. Am. Med. Assoc.*, 270, 841, 1993.

74. Miller, J. Z., Smith, D. L., Flora, L., Slemenda, C., Jiang, X., and Johnston, C. C., Calcium absorption from calcium carbonate and a new form of calcium (CCM) in healthy male and female adolescents, *Am. J. Clin. Nutr.*, 48, 1291, 1988.

75. Gleerup, A., Rossander-Hulten, L., Gramatkovski, E., and Hallberg, L. Iron absorption from the whole diet: comparison of the effect of two different distributions of daily calcium intake, *Am. J. Clin. Nutr.*, 61, 97, 1995.

76. Cook, J. D., Dassenko, S. A., and Whittaker, P., Calcium supplementation: effect on iron absorption, *Am. J. Clin. Nutr.*, 53, 106, 1991.

77. Heaney, R. P., Optimal calcium intake, *J. Am. Med. Assoc.*, 274, 1012, 1995.

78. Davies, K. J. A., Maguire, J. J., Brooks, G. A., Dallman, P. R., and Packer, L., Muscle mitochondrial bioenergetics, oxygen supply, and work capacity during dietary iron deficiency and repletion, *Am. J. Physiol.*, 242, E418, 1982.

79. Cook, J. D., Dassenko, S. A., and Lynch, S. R., Assessment of the role of nonheme-iron availability in iron balance, *Am. J. Clin. Nutr.*, 54, 717, 1991.

80. Gavin, M. W., McCarthy, D. M., and Garry, P. J., Evidence that iron stores regulate iron absorption — a setpoint theory, *Am. J. Clin. Nutr.*, 59, 1376, 1994.

81. Cook. J. D., Adaptation in iron metabolism, *Am. J. Clin. Nutr.*, 51, 301, 1990.

82. Hallberg, L. and Rossander-Hultén, L., Iron requirements in menstruating women, *Am. J. Clin. Nutr.*, 54, 1047, 1991.

83. Fairbanks, V. F., Iron, in *Modern Nutrition In Health and Disease*, Shils, M.E., Olson, J. A. and Shike, M., (Eds.), 8th ed., Lea & Febiger, Philadelphia, 1994, 185.

84. Monsen, E. R. and Balintfy, J. L., Calculating dietary iron bioavailability: refinement and computerization, *J. Am. Diet. Assoc.*, 80, 307, 1982.

85. Monsen, E. R., Hallberg, L., Layrisse, M., Hegsted, D. M., Cook. J. D., Mertz, W., and Finch, C. A., Estimation of available dietary iron, *Am. J. Clin. Nutr.*, 31, 134, 1978.

86. Cook, J. D. and Monsen, E. R., Food iron absorption in human subjects. III. Comparison of the effect of animal proteins on nonheme iron absorption, *Am. J. Clin. Nutr.*, 29, 859, 1976.

87. Morck, T. A., Lynch, S. R., and Cook, J. D., Inhibition of food iron absorption by coffee, *Am. J. Clin. Nutr.*, 37, 416, 1983.

88. Balaban, E. P., Cox, J. V., Snell, P., Vaughan, R. H., and Frenkel, E. P., The frequency of anemia and iron deficiency in the runner, *Med. Sci. Sports Exerc.*, 21, 643, 1989.

89. Williford, H. N., Olson, M. S., Keith, R. E., Barksdale, J. M., Blessing, D. L., Wang, N., and Preston, P., Iron status in women aerobic dance instructors, *Int. J. Sport Nutr.*, 3, 387, 1993.

90. Lampe, J. W., Slavin, J. L., and Apple, F. S., Poor iron status of women runners training for a marathon, *Int. J. Sports Med.*, 7, 111, 1986.

91. Diehl, D. M., Lohman, T. G., Smith, S. C., and Kertzer, R., Effects of physical training and competition on the iron status of female field hockey players, *Int. J. Sports Med.*, 7, 264, 1986.

92. Nickerson, H. J., Holubets, M. C., Weiler, B. R., Haas, R. G., Schwartz, S., and Ellefson, M. E., Causes of iron deficiency in adolescent athletes, *J. Pediatr.*, 114, 675, 1989.

93. Rowland, T. W., Stagg, L., and Kelleher, J. F., Iron deficiency in adolescent girls, *J. Adol. Health*, 12, 22, 1991.

94. Telford, R. D., Cunningham, R. B., Deakin, V., and Kerr, D. A., Iron status and diet in athletes, *Med. Sci. Sports Exerc.*, 25, 796, 1993.

95. Risser, W. L., Lee, E. J., Poindexter, H. B. W., West, M. S., Pivarnik, J. M., Risser, J. M. H., and Hickson, J. F., Iron deficiency in female athletes: its prevalence and impact on performance, *Med. Sci. Sports Exerc.*, 20, 116, 1988.

96. Snyder, A. C., Dvorak, L. L., and Roepke, J. B., Influence of dietary iron source on measures of iron status among female runners, *Med. Sci. Sports Exerc.*, 21, 7, 1989.

97. van Erp Baart, A. M. J., Saris, W. H. M., Binkhorst, R. A., Vos, J. A., and Elvers, J. W. H., Nationwide survey on nutritional habits in elite athletes, Part II. Mineral and vitamin intake, *Int. J. Sport Nutr.*, 10, S11, 1989.

98. Cook, J. D. and Finch, C. A., Assessing iron status of a population, *Am. J. Clin. Nutr.*, 32, 2115, 1979.

99. Harris, S. S., Helping active women avoid anemia, *Phys. Sportsmed.*, 23, 35, 1995.

100. Kim, I., Yetley, E. A., and Calvo, M. S., Variations in iron-status measures during the menstrual cycle, *Am. J. Clin. Nutr.*, 58, 705, 1993.

101. Dickson, D. N., Wilkinson, R. L., and Noakes, T. D., Effects of ultra-marathon training and racing on hematologic parameters and serum ferritin levels in well-trained athletes, *Int. J. Sports Med.*, 3, 111, 1982.

102. Lampe, J. W., Slavin, J. L., and Apple, F. S., Iron status of active women and the effect of running a marathon on bowel function and gastrointestinal blood loss, *Int. J. Sport Med.*, 12, 173, 1991.

103. Miller, B. J., Pate, R. R., and Burgess, W., Foot impact force intravascular hemolysis during distance running, *Int. J. Sports Med.*, 9, 56, 1988.

104. Lamanca, J. J., Haymes, E. M., Daly, J. A., Moffatt, R. J., and Waller, M. F., Sweat iron loss of male and female runners during exercise, *Int. J. Sports Med.*, 9, 52, 1988.

105. Bothwell, T. H., Overview and mechanisms of iron regulation, *Nutr. Rev.*, 53, 237, 1995.

106. Hunt, J. R., Gallagher, S. K., and Johnson, L. K., Effect of ascorbic acid on apparent iron absorption by women with low iron stores, *Am. J. Clin. Nutr.*, 59, 1381, 1994.

107. Fetherman, D. L., Shock, M. M., Ishee, J. H., and Lowe, R. C., Dietary iron status of female runners, *Int. J. Sport Nutr.*, 5, 81, 1995.

108. Manore, M. M., Besenfelder, P. D., Wells, C. L., Carroll, S. S., and Hooker. S. P., Nutrient intakes and iron status in female long-distance runners during training, *J. Am. Diet. Assoc.*, 89, 257, 1989.

109. Newhouse, I. J., Clement, D. B., Taunton, J. E., and McKenzie, D. C., The effects of prelatent/latent iron deficiency on physical work capacity, *Med. Sci. Sports Exerc.*, 21, 263, 1989.

110. Weight, L. M., Jacobs, P., and Noakes, T. D., Dietary iron deficiency and sports anaemia, *Br. J. Nutr.*, 68, 253, 1992.

111. Food and Nutrition Board, National Research Council, *Recommended Dietary Allowances*, 10th ed., National Academy Press, Washington, D.C., 1989, 199.

112. Reggiani, E., Arras, G. B., Trabacca, S., Senarega, D., and Chiodini, G., Nutritional status and body composition of adolescent female gymnasts, *J. Sports Med.*, 29, 285, 1989.

113. Kirchner, E. M., Lewis, R. D., and O'Connor, P. J., Bone mineral density and dietary intake of female college gymnasts, *Med. Sci. Sports Exerc.*, 27, 543, 1995.

114. Moffatt, R. J., Dietary status of elite female high school gymnasts: inadequacy of vitamin and mineral intake, *J. Am. Diet. Assoc.*, 84, 1361, 1984.

115. Loosli, A. R., Benson, J., Gillien, D. M., and Bourdet, K., Nutrition habits and knowledge in competitive adolescent female gymnasts, *Phys. Sportsmed.*, 14, 118, 1986.

116. Benardot, D., Schwarz, M., and Heller, D. W., Nutrient intake in young, highly competitive gymnasts, *J. Am. Diet. Assoc.*, 89, 401, 1989.

117. Alaimo, K., McDowell, M. A., Briefel, R. R., Bischof, A. M., Caughman, C. R., Loria, C. M., and Johnson, C. L., Dietary Intake of vitamins, minerals, and fiber of persons ages 2 months and over in the United States: Third National Health and Nutrition Examination Survey, Phase 1, 1988-1991, Advance data from vital and health statistics; no 258, Hyattsville, Maryland, National Center for Health Statistics, 1994.

118. McDowell, M.A., Briefel, R. R., Alaimo, K., Bischof, A. M., Caughman, C. R., Carroll, M. D., Loria, C. M., and Johnson, C. L., Energy and macronutrient intakes of persons ages 2 months and over in the United States:Third National Health and Nutrition Examination Survey, Phase 1, 1988-1991, Advance data from vital and health statistics, No. 255, Hyattsville, Maryland, National Center for Health Statistics, 1994.

119. Evers, C. L., Dietary intake and symptoms of anorexia nervosa in female university dancers, *J. Am. Diet. Assoc.*, 87, 66, 1987.

120. Cohen, J. L., Potosnak, L., Frank, O., and Baker, H., A nutritional and hematologic assessment of elite ballet dancers, *Phys. Sportsmed.*, 13, 43, 1985.

121. Donovan, U. M. and Gibson, R. S., Iron and zinc status of young women aged 14 to 19 years consuming vegetarian and omnivorous diets, *J. Am. Coll. Nutr.*, 14, 463, 1995.

122. Klingshirn, L. A., Pate, R. R., Bourque, S. P., Davis, J. M., and Sargent, R. G., Effect of iron supplementation on endurance capacity in iron-depleted female runners, *Med. Sci. Sports Exerc.*, 24, 819, 1992.

123. Fogelholm, M., Jaakkola, L., and Lampisjärvi, T., Effects of iron supplementation in female athletes with low serum ferritin concentration, *Int. J. Sports Med.*, 13, 158, 1992.

124. Rowland, T. W., Deisroth, M. B., Green, G. M., and Kelleher, J. F., The effect of iron therapy on the exercise capacity of nonanemic iron-deficient adolecent runners. *Am. J. Disease Child.*, 142, 165, 1988.

125. Telford, R. D., Bunney, C. J., Catchpole, E. A., Catchpole, W. R., Deakin, V., Gray, B., Hahn, A. G., and Kerr, D. A., Plasma ferritin concentration and physical work capacity in athletes, *Int. J. Sport Nutr.*, 2, 335, 1992.

126. Loosli, A. R., unpublished data, 1995.

127. Difiori, J. P. and Puffer, J. C., Track and field, in *Sports Medicine Secrets*, Mellion, M. B.,(Ed.), Hanley & Belfus, Philadelphia, 1994, 379.

128. Nieman, D. C., Gates, J. R., Butler, J. V., Pollett, L. M., Dietrich, S. J., and Lutz, R. D., Supplementation patterns in marathon runners, *J. Am. Diet. Assoc.*, 89, 1615, 1989.

129. Khoo, C. S., Rawson, N. E., Robinson, M. L., and Stevenson, R. J., Nutrient intake and eating habits of triathletes, *Ann. Sports Med.*, 3, 144, 1987.

130. Singh, A., Evans, P., Gallagher, K. L., and Deuster, P. A., Dietary intakes and biochemical profiles of nutritional status of ultramarathoners, *Med. Sci. Sports Exerc.*, 25, 328, 1993.

131. Deuster, P. A., Kyle, S. B., Moser, P. B., Vigersky, R. A., Singh, A., and Schoomaker, E. B., Nutritional intakes and status of highly trained amenorrheic and eumenorrheic women runners, *Fert. Steril.*, 46, 636, 1986.

132. Viteri, F. E., Xunian, L., Tolomei, K., and Martín, A., True absorption and retention of supplemental iron is more efficient when iron is administered every three days rather than daily to iron-normal and iron-deficient rats, *J. Nutr.*, 125, 82, 1995.

133. Wright, A. J. A. and Southon, S., The effectiveness of various iron-supplementation regimens in improving the Fe status of anaemic rats, *Br. J. Nutr.*, 63, 579, 1990.

134. Schultink, W., Gross, R., Gliwitzki, M., Karyadi, D., and Matulessi, P., Effect of daily vs. twice weekly iron supplementation in Indonesian preschool children with low iron status, *Am. J. Clin. Nutr.*, 61, 111, 1995.

135. Stephenson, L. S., Possible new developments in community control of iron-deficiency anemia, *Nutr. Rev.*, 53, 23, 1995.

136. Cook, J. D. and Reddy, M. B., Efficacy of weekly compared with daily iron supplementation, *Am. J. Clin. Nutr.*, 62, 117, 1995.

137. Yadrick, M. K., Kenney, M. A., and Winterfeldt, E. A., Iron, copper, and zinc status: response to supplementation with zinc or zinc and iron in adult females, *Am. J. Clin. Nutr.*, 49, 145, 1989.

138. Solomons, N. W., Competitive interaction of iron and zinc in the diet:consequences for human nutrition, *J. Nutr.*, 116, 927, 1986.

139. Sandstrom, B., Davidsson, L., Cederblad, A., and Lonnerdal, B. Oral iron, dietary ligands and zinc absorption, *J. Nutr.*, 115, 411, 1985.

140. King, J. C. and Keen, C. L., Zinc, in *Modern Nutrition in Health and Disease*, Shils, M. E., Olson, J. A., and Shike, M., (Eds.), 8th ed., Lea & Febiger, Philadelphia, 1994, 214.

141. Food and Nutrition Board, National Research Council, *Recommended Dietary Allowances*, 10th ed., National Academy Press, Washington, D.C., 1989, 209.

142. Mares-Perlman, J. A., Subar, A. F., Block, G., Greger, J. L., and Luby, M. H., Zinc intake and sources in the US adult population: 1976-1980, *J. Am. Coll. Nutr.*, 14, 349, 1995.

143. Yokoi, K., Alcock, N. W., and Sandstead, H. H., Iron and zinc nutriture of premenopausal women: Associations of diet with serum ferritin and plasma zinc disappearance and of serum ferritin with plasma zinc and plasma zinc disappearance, *J. Lab. Clin. Med.*, 124, 852, 1994.

144. Hunt, J. R., Gallagher, S. K., Johnson, L. K., and Lykken, G. I., High-versus low-meat diets:effects on zinc absorption, iron status, and calcium, copper, iron, magnesium, manganese, nitrogen, phosphorus, and zinc balance in postmenopausal women, *Am. J. Clin. Nutr.*, 62, 621, 1995.

145. Deuster, P. A., Day, B. A., Singh, A., Douglass, L., and Moser-Veillon, P. B., Zinc status of highly trained women runners and untrained women, *Am. J. Clin. Nutr.*, 49, 1295, 1989.

146. Singh, A., Deuster, P. A., and Moser, P. B., Zinc and copper status of women by physical activity and menstrual status, *J. Sports Med. Phys. Fitness*, 30, 29, 1990.

147. Haralambie, G., Serum zinc in athletes in training, *Int. J. Sports Med.*, 2, 135, 1981.

148. Tipton, K., Green, N. R., Haymes, E. M., and Waller, M., Zinc loss in sweat of athletes exercising in hot and neutral temperatures, *Int. J. Sport Nutr.*, 3, 261, 1993.

149. Couzy, F., Lafargue, P., and Guezennec, C. Y., Zinc metabolism in the athlete: influence of training, nutrition and other factors, *Int. J. Sports Med.*, 11, 263, 1990.

150. Dolev, E., Burstein, R., Lubin, F., Wishnizer, R., Chetrit, A., Shefi, M., and Deuster, P. A., Interpretation of zinc status indicators in a strenuously exercising population, *J. Am. Diet. Assoc.*, 95, 482, 1995.

151. Nowak, R. K., Knudsen, K. S., and Schulz, L. O., Body composition and nutrient intakes of college men and women basketball players, *J. Am. Diet. Assoc.*, 88, 575, 1988.

Chapter 5

WATER AND ELECTROLYTES

CONTENTS

I. INTRODUCTION

After oxygen, water is the most important nutrient needed by the body. We can live for days, even weeks, without food, but we can survive only 5 to 10 days, at most, without water.

Water plays a vital role in an athlete's performance. One crucial function is the regulation of body temperature. During exercise in the heat, large amounts of water may be lost through sweat as the body attempts to maintain normal body temperature. Water must be consumed regularly and in sufficient amounts to ensure normal body functions and thermal regulation. Failure to replace water loss results in dehydration, which can impair performance. The focus of this chapter is on the role of water and electrolytes in athletic performance.

II. FUNCTIONS OF WATER

Water performs many distinct and vital functions. In the body, water acts as:

- A solvent for products of digestion
- A medium for digestion, absorption, metabolism, secretion and excretion
- A component of all body cells, giving structure and form to the body
- A temperature regulator
- A lubricant surrounding the joints, heart, and intestines
- A cushion for the brain and spinal cord

Water is the largest component of the body, representing 45 to 70% of body weight.[1] Total body water is determined largely by body composition; muscle tissue is about 75% water while fat tissue is about 20% water. The higher the percentage of muscle mass, the higher the percentage of water in the body. Women contain less muscle mass than men which explains why 50% of a woman's body weight is water, compared to 60% for men. Obese individuals have a relatively lower total body water (40%) by virtue of a greater amount of fat tissue.

III. RECOMMENDATIONS AND SOURCES

The requirement for water as suggested by the Committee on the Recommended Dietary Allowances is 1 ml/kcal of energy expenditure for adults under normal conditions of energy expenditure and environmental exposure.[2] For the female who expends 2200 kcal/d, this equals about 1500 to 2000 ml (48–64 oz) of water a day. This recommendation may be increased to 1.5 ml/kcal to cover variations in activity level, sweating, and solute load.[2]

Water is taken into the body by direct consumption: it is derived from (1) fluids, (2) solid foods, and (3) the oxidation of food. Approximately two thirds of daily water intake is in the form of beverages such as water, tea, coffee, milk, and soda. The remainder comes from food. Nearly all foods contain water, especially fruits and vegetables which contain up to 95% water.

Many meats and cheese contain around 50% water, while breads contain approximately 35% water. The metabolism of 100 g of protein, carbohydrate, and fat produces approximately 40, 55, and 107 g of water, respectively.

IV. DISTRIBUTION OF WATER IN THE BODY

Total body water is distributed between two main fluid compartments: the intracellular compartment and the extracellular compartment. Excellular fluid includes interstitial fluid, plasma, cerebrospinal fluid, intraocular fluid, and the fluid in the gastrointestinal tract.[3] Of a total fluid volume of about 40 liters, 15 liters are extracellular (3 liters in the blood plasma), and the remaining 25 liters are intracellular (Figure 5.1).[3] Although the extracellular fluid is less than half that of the intracellular fluid, it is of great importance, since it is the extracellular fluid that supplies the cells with nutrients and other substances needed for cellular function.

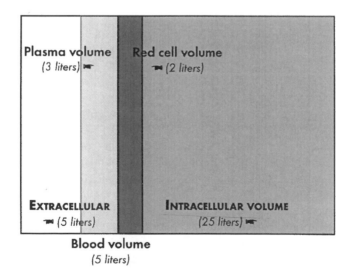

Blood volume
(5 liters)

FIGURE 5.1   Diagram of the body fluids, showing the extracellular fluid volume, intracellular fluid volume, blood volume, and total body fluids. From Guyton, A. C., *Human Physiology and Mechanisms of Disease,* 5th ed., W. B. Saunders Company, Philadelphia, 1992, 197. With permission.

Water balance is maintained when fluid intake equals fluid output. Normally, the average adult loses about 2 liters of water a day in urine, sweat, feces, and evaporation through the lungs.[3] However, water loss varies greatly from person to person depending on a number of factors. For example, fecal losses can range from 100 ml/d on a normal varied diet to 3 liters or more during diarrhea. Urine volume can vary depending on fluid intake, diet, exercise, and temperature. At a temperature of 20°C (68°F), approximately 1400 ml of water is lost in urine. However, during prolonged heavy exercise in hot weather, only 500 ml of water is lost in urine.[3]

Of all potential routes for water loss during exercise, sweating is the most significant.[4] The amount of body fluid lost as sweat can vary greatly and depends on the individual, the intensity of exercise, and the environmental temperature and humidity. Under normal temperatures, about 1 liter of water is lost in sweat. However, during prolonged strenuous exercise in the heat, sweat rates of 1.5 to 2 l/h are common,[5] and daily losses as high as 3.7 l/h have been reported.[6]

Normally, body heat is dissipated by convection and radiation, but when large amounts of metabolic heat are produced, such as during strenuous exercise, these systems are not adequate and sweating becomes the primary cooling system. It is important that the athlete understand the role of sweating in maintaining body temperature. Water must be consumed regularly and in sufficient amounts to ensure proper hydration. Failure to replace water loss results in dehydration, which can cause decrements in performance.

According to Brouns et al.,[7] under some circumstances, sweat response in females may be different from that in males. In high humidity, females have lower sweat rates. Moreover, compared to males, females have a higher sweat efficiency and higher sweat onset threshold as well as higher sweat sodium levels.[5]

V. DEHYDRATION AND EXERCISE

Dehydration and hypohydration are two terms often used to describe a decrease in body water. According to Sawka,[1] hypohydration refers to a body water deficit, whereas the more common term, dehydration, refers to the dynamic loss of body water or the transition from euhydration to hypohydration. In practice, the two terms are often used interchangeably.

The physiological effects of dehydration on exercise performance have been extensively studied and several excellent reviews have been written.[1,8–10] A water loss of only 1% body weight impairs thermoregulation leading to a decrease in physical work capacity. At 3 to 5% water loss, the body's ability to efficiently utilize oxygen is impaired; and at 7% loss, collapse is likely (Figure 5.2). Even small deficits have adverse effects on performance through elevated heart rate, reduced sweat rates, and increased body core temperature.[11] Thus, adequate fluid intake during exercise is critical to health and performance.

Unfortunately, many athletes do not know how serious dehydration can be or what to do about it.[8] For example, 86% of college athletes surveyed by Grandjean et al.[12] knew that adequate water intake before, during, and after practice helps to prevent dehydration, however, 53% did not know how much water to consume. On the other hand, sports nutritionists are very aware that athletes need to drink more water than thirst demands when training or competing in hot environments.[13]

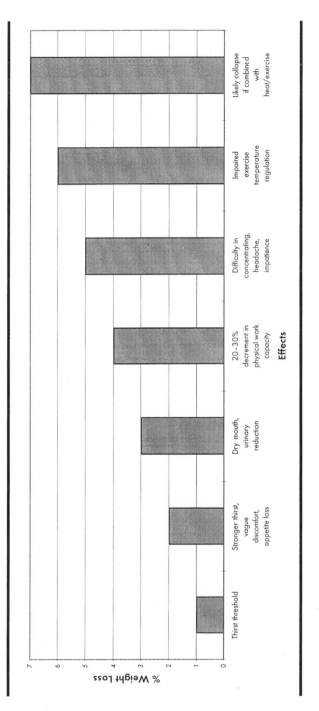

FIGURE 5.2 Adverse Effects of Dehydration. (From Greenleaf, J. E. and Harrison, M. H., Water and electrolytes, in *Nutrition and Aerobic Exercise*, Layman, D. K. (Ed.), American Chemical Society, Washington, D.C., 1986, 115. With permission.)

A. INVOLUNTARY DEHYDRATION

Humans will voluntarily restrict fluid intake, and thus, not adequately replace water. This condition, known as involuntary dehydration, occurs primarily in individuals when they are exposed to various stresses including environmental heat and cold, altitude, water immersion, and exercise.[9] The more stressful the situation, the greater is the level of dehydration and the longer it takes to replace lost fluids.[8]

Physiological, psychological, and environmental factors influence fluid consumption.[14] Two important considerations are temperature and taste. Boulze et al.[15] reported that during induced dehydration, subjects consumed the most when water temperature was 15°C (59°F) and drank less when warmer or cooler water was offered. Hubbard et al.[16] also found that cooling and flavoring water decreased the extent of involuntary dehydration during exercise in the heat.

One of the main reasons for the growth and success of the sports drink industry is taste. Although athletes can get the fluids they need from drinking plain water, many prefer the taste of sports drinks. Thus, a major benefit of sports drinks is the prevention of hypohydration due to an increase in voluntary intake of fluids.

Dehydration during exercise can be rapid (acute) or gradual (chronic). Acute dehydration can occur in a matter of hours and is commonly seen in marathon runners and triathletes. An example of acute dehydration was observed in Swiss runner Gabriela Anderson-Schiess who nearly collapsed from heat exhaustion during the women's marathon at the 1984 Olympic summer games. Acute dehydration can be prevented when fluids are consumed before, during, and after training or competition.

Chronic dehydration is less obvious and occurs when athletes such as football, soccer, or basketball players train daily in hot environments and do not drink enough fluids to adequately rehydrate. To ensure adequate fluid replacement, body weight should be measured before and after training sessions. For every pound lost, the athlete should drink 500 ml (16 oz) of fluid.[17] If weight is not within 0.45 to 0.9 kg (1 to 2 lb) of the previous day's weight, additional fluids should be consumed before exercising.[17]

B. INTENTIONAL DEHYDRATION

While most athletes want to avoid dehydration, some athletes, such as wrestlers, weight lifters, and light-weight rowers, purposely dehydrate themselves to reach a desired weight class. Dancers, figure skaters, and body builders are also known to intentionally dehydrate in an effort to maintain a low body weight or to improve appearance prior to competition.[18] Dehydration techniques used for rapid weight reduction include fluid restriction, exercising in a rubber or plastic suit, taking a sauna, and use of laxatives and/or diuretics.[19] In a study by Kleiner et al.,[20] male and female bodybuilders reported severe fluid restrictions, and dehydrating practices such as riding stationary bicycles in a sauna while wearing a rubberized suit, and expectorating.

Strumi and Rutecki[21] recently reported on a professional bodybuilder who collapsed shortly after the start of a professional bodybuilding competition. Diagnosis revealed hyperkalemia due to the use of potassium-sparing diuretics and potassium supplements. Three days before competition, the bodybuilder had consumed only 1500 ml (48 oz) of water and one bowl of steamed rice. He had not urinated for 18 h and had lost approximately 9 kg (20 lb) over the 3-day period. This study illustrates how life-threatening fluid and calorie restriction can be, especially in combination with drugs and dietary supplements.

Many coaches and athletes do not recognize the compromising effects of moderate dehydration. Houston et al.[22] showed significant decreases in muscle glycogen levels and dynamic strength in four college wrestlers who decreased body weight by 8% over a 4-day period through food and fluid restriction. In another study, Burge et al.[23] examined the effect of rapid dehydration and rehydration on performance and physiological function during high intensity rowing in elite lightweight rowers. Athletes used a combination of food and fluid restriction and low intensity exercise in a sweatsuit to reduce body weight. Results of the study indicated that dehydration caused a significant decrease in the ability to sustain work at high intensity. The authors attributed these findings to lowered plasma volume and decreased muscle glycogen utilization.

VI. GUIDELINES FOR OPTIMAL FLUID REPLACEMENT

The process of rehydration depends on both gastric emptying and intestinal absorption.[24] Several factors influence the rate of gastric emptying, including volume, type of drink, temperature, and osmolality.[25] Gastric emptying increases in direct proportion to the volume of fluid consumed. Larger volumes (up to 600 ml) empty more rapidly from the stomach, although smaller amounts, 150 to 250 ml, at 10 to 15 min intervals may be more practical for the athlete.[26]

As the carbohydrate content of a beverage increases, its osmolality increases, reducing the rate of gastric emptying.[24] Studies show that commercial sport beverages containing 6 to 8% carbohydrate in the form of glucose, glucose polymers, or sucrose are absorbed quickly from the stomach and help maintain blood glucose levels during exercise.[27,28] However, beverages that exceed 10% carbohydrate may impair gastric emptying and fluid replacement, particularly during prolonged exercise in the heat.[29] Likewise, drinks containing fructose as the primary carbohydrate source have been associated with gastric distress, diarrhea, and nausea in some athletes, and thus may limit performance.[30]

The ideal fluid replacement beverage depends on the duration and intensity of exercise, the environmental temperature, and the athlete. Guidelines for optimal replacement beverages for different athletic events are presented in Table 5.1. For most athletes who are exercising for 1 hour or less in a moderate temperature, cool water is the best choice. The major concern in events lasting less than 1 hour is the rise in body temperature.[24] According to Gisolfi and Duchman,[24] there is little need to replace sodium under these circumstances because sweat losses generally do not exceed 2 to 3 l/h. Furthermore, Gisolfi and Duchman[24] do not recommend the addition of carbohydrate to an oral solution during exercise less than 1 hour because of the possible delay in gastric emptying. However, there is some evidence that a carbohydrate beverage will enhance performance. Below et al.[31] demonstrated that both water and a 6% carbohydrate-electrolyte solution, independently, improved performance during 1 hour of cycling at 80% VO_{2max}.

During endurance events lasting longer than 90 min of continuous effort, the best fluid replacement beverage is one that tastes good, does not cause gastric upset, provides a source of carbohdyrate for energy, and delays the onset of dehydration.[32] The addition of electrolytes can also enhance fluid intake and absorption and can delay fatigue during exercise.[7,24] Moreover, it has been shown that providing a carbohydrate-electrolyte beverage during prolonged heavy exercise extends endurance capacity by delaying muscle glycogen depletion.[33,34]

VII. GLYCEROL

In recent years, glycerol has gained popularity as an effective way to "hyperhydrate" prior to training and competition. Glycerol is a clear, sweet, syrupy liquid found naturally in many foods and is also added to many processed foods. Research has examined the effects of glycerol in preventing dehydration and enhancing endurance performance.[35-37]

Glycerol's chemical properties are said to be suitable for enhancing an athlete's hydration status. It is rapidly absorbed when taken orally and evenly distributed throughout body fluids.

Research on the beneficial effects of glycerol presently is limited and somewhat conflicting. Data showed that subjects who consumed a glycerol solution 2.5 hours before exercise in the heat had less urine output, lower body temperature, and increased sweat rate compared to subjects who drank just water.[35] However, research by Murray et al.[36] found no indication of hyperhydration in subjects consuming a glycerol solution during exercise. Differences in the subjects, dosage, and timing may account for the discrepancies.

Two different mechanisms have been reported for glycerol's effect on body fluid regulation.[35,37] The first is that glycerol initially expands total body water by increasing the volume of the interstitial fluid and intracellular fluid with little effect on plasma volume. The excess water in the extravascular space is readily available to maintain plasma volume, thereby increasing sweat rate and reducing the rise in body temperature during exercise and thermal stress.

TABLE 5.1   Recommended Guidelines for Optimal Fluid Replacement

Event Time	<1 hour	1 to 3 hours	>3 hours	Recovery
	80 to 130% Vo₂Max	*60 to 90% Vo₂Max*	*30 to 70% Vo₂Max*	
Primary concerns	To prevent excessive rise in core body temperature	For fluid and carbohydrate provision	Fluid, energy, and electrolyte provision	Glycogen resynthesis, fluid replacement and sodium replacement
Pre-event	300 to 500 ml of a 6 to 10% carbohydrate beverage	300 to 500 ml of water	300 to 500 ml of water	
During exercise	500 to 1,000 ml cool water	800 to 1,600 ml/h of a cool 6 to 8% carbohydrate beverage	500 to 1,000 ml/h of a cool 6 to 8% carbohydrate beverage	
Electrolyte replacement	No need to replace electrolytes such as sodium, chloride, or potassium	10 to 20 mEq/l of sodium and chloride to promote carbohydrate and fluid absorption	20 to 30 mEq of sodium and chloride to promote carbohydrate and fluid absorption	30 to 40 mEq of sodium and chloride to enhance fluid replacement

Adapted from Gisolfi, C. V. and Duchman, S. M. Guidelines for optimal replacement beverages for different athletic events, *Med. Sci. Sports Exerc.*, 24, 679, 1992.

The second theory for enhanced water retention may be the osmotic effects of glycerol on antidiuretic hormone. Freund et al.[37] proposed that antidiuretic hormone may be partly responsible for glycerol's effectiveness in improving fluid retention. Antidiuretic hormone is produced by the pituitary gland in response to dehydration. This hormone stimulates the kidneys to reabsorb more water and thus excrete less water. According to Freund et al.,[37] even small changes in antidiuretic hormone levels can have marked effects on urine flow and osmolarity.

Whether glycerol can improve performance is unclear. Montner et al.[38] compared the effects of prehydration with equal volumes of water (25 ml/kg) and a glycerol and water solution (1.2 g/kg bw) on endurance time, rectal temperature, hydration status, and heart rate during cycling. Compared with water, glycerol was associated with significantly longer endurance times (94 min vs. 77 min). Subjects who drank the glycerol solution had lower body temperature and lower heart rate which the authors attributed to enhanced expansion of plasma volume. Further research is needed to confirm this observation.

Oral doses of glycerol up to 1 g per kg of body weight every 6 hours appear to be safe.[35] However, as with any substance, glycerol may be tolerated differently by each athlete. Headaches, bloating, nausea, vomiting, and dizziness have been reported with the use of glycerol.[36]

VIII. ELECTROLYTES

Electrolytes are substances which, in water, are able to conduct an electrical current. These include the minerals sodium, chloride, and potassium. Sodium and chloride are found primarily in the extracellular fluids, while potassium is located mainly in the intracellular fluids. The major function of electrolytes is to control and maintain the regulation of body water distribution between the various fluid compartments. Electrolytes are also important for muscle contraction and transmission of nerve impulses.

One of the questions frequently asked by coaches and athletes is whether an athlete should replace electrolytes that may be lost through sweat. Generally, the need to replace lost body fluid is much greater than any immediate demands for electrolytes.[26]

Compared with other body fluids, sweat is hypotonic. Table 5.2 shows the composition of sweat in relation to that of plasma and muscle. Sodium and chloride are the major ions in sweat and blood. However, the ionic concentration of sweat can vary substantially between individuals and is greatly influenced by the rate of sweat, the person's state of heat acclimatization, and the dietary intake of electrolytes.[26]

A. SODIUM

Sodium helps regulate body fluids and helps maintain normal blood volume. Sodium is also needed for the normal function of nerves and muscles.

TABLE 5.2   Electrolyte Concentrations and Osmolality in Sweat, Muscle, and Plasma (mmol/l)

	Sodium (Na)	Chloride (Cl)	Potassium (K)	Magnesium (Mg)	Osmolarity (mOsmol/l)
Sweat	40–60	30–50	4–5	1.5–5	80–185
Plasma	140	101	4	1.5	302
Muscle	9	9	162	31	302

Adapted from Costill, D. L. and Miller, J. M., Nutrition for endurance sport: carbohydrate and fluid balance. *Int. J. Sports Med.,* 1, 2, 1980.

Of all the electrolytes, sodium is the one most affected by physical exercise. Under extreme conditions, athletes who sweat profusely, who are not acclimated to the heat, or who have low sodium intakes may experience heat cramps or exhaustion due to sodium depletion.[39] Thus, certain athletes may need to increase their intake of foods higher in sodium or consume a fluid replacement beverage with added sodium.

Studies have shown that rehydration during and after exercise in the heat occurs more rapidly when sodium is added to fluids.[40-42] Nose et al.[40] found that subjects rehydrating with water and sodium restored more lost fluid after exercise than water alone. Maughan and Leiper[42] recently studied the effects of four test drinks containing different amounts of sodium on rehydration after exercise. Sodium salts were added to give a sodium concentration of 2, 25, 52, and 100 mmol/l, respectively. Results showed that urine volume was inversely proportional to the sodium content of the drinks consumed. This study demonstrates that the addition of sodium to fluids consumed after exercise is beneficial in restoring fluid balance.

On the other hand, drinking large amounts of plain water with very little sodium to compensate for sweat loss may induce hyponatremia (serum sodium concentrations below 130 mmol/l).[43] Hyponatremia has been observed during ultraendurance events such as 50-mile runs and triathlons.[44-46] Symptoms include lethargy, drowsiness, muscle weakness, muscle cramping, and mental confusion. Fortunately, this condition is not common in the majority of athletes.

1. Requirements

For most athletes, a normal diet offers enough sodium for optimal performance. The average American consumes between 4,000 to 6,000 mg of sodium per day. Sodium intakes of endurance runners and triathletes reportedly ranged from 2,260 to 4,425 mg/d.[47]

Because every athlete is different, the exact amount of sodium required for optimal health and performance is not known. Health experts recommend limiting the amount of sodium to 2,400 mg/d. Sodium occurs naturally in many foods, but the biggest single source of sodium in most people's diets is salt added to foods. One teaspoon of salt contains 2,325 mg. Sodium is also added to many foods and beverages. Processed foods generally are high in sodium. The sodium content of sports drinks is between 10 to 25 mmol/l. Most soft drinks contain very little sodium, less than 4 mmol/l.[41]

B. POTASSIUM

Potassium assists in muscular contraction and nerve conduction and in maintaining fluid and electrolyte balance in body cells. It also plays an important role in the transport of glucose across cell membrances and the storage of glycogen.

Potassium balance is regulated by dietary intake, exchange between the intracellular and extracellular fluid compartments, and excretion or retention by the kidneys.[48] Approximately 40 mEq of potassium is excreted in a liter of urine, so changes in renal function and urine output will have an effect on potassium balance.[48]

Potassium is lost from the body in the urine and to a lesser degree, in gastrointestinal secretions. The most frequent cause of potassium deficiency is excess loss, usually through the alimentary tract or the kidneys.[49]

For most athletes, including those performing in ultraendurance events in the heat, a potassium deficiency is not a concern because potassium losses in sweat are low. However, athletes who have recently suffered severe diarrhea or vomiting, or who use diuretics, may risk potassium deficiency.

In healthy individuals, a dietary deficiency of potassium is unlikely, although low potassium intakes can occur if fresh fruits and vegetables are lacking in the diet.

1. Requirements

The National Research Council's RDA for potassium is 40 to 50 mEq/d (1,600 to 2,000 mg/d).[49] Potassium is widely distributed in foods, with the richest sources being fresh fruits, vegetables, fresh meats, and dairy products. A good food source of potassium provides at least 50 mEq (200 mg) per serving.

IX. CONCLUSIONS

Water is an important nutrient for the athlete. It must be consumed regularly and in sufficient amounts to ensure normal functioning of the body and thermal regulation. Failure to replace water loss results in dehydration which can impair performance.

All athletes need to be aware of the harmful effects of heat, humidity, and dehydration. During strenuous prolonged exercise, some athletes can lose up to 3 liters of sweat per hour. Athletes should consume 500 ml fluid 2 hours before exercise followed by another 500 ml 15 to 20 min before exercise and

118 to 177 ml of fluid every 10 to 15 min during exercise. Specific fluid requirements for different athletic events were briefly reviewed.

Sodium is the electrolyte most affected by physical exercise. But in most cases, the athlete's typical diet provides enough sodium, potassium, and other electrolytes to replace sweat losses.

REFERENCES

1. Sawka, M. N., Physiological consequences of hypohydration: exercise performance and thermoregulation, *Med. Sci. Sports Exerc.*, 24, 657, 1992.
2. Food and Nutrition Board, National Research Council, *Recommended Dietary Allowances*, 10th ed., National Academy Press Washington, D.C., 1989, 252.
3. Guyton, A. C., *Human Physiology and Mechanisms of Disease*, W. B. Saunders Company, 5th ed., Philadelphia, 1992.
4. Wright, E. D., Fluid and electrolyte requirements during exercise, *J. Clin. Nutr.*, 7, 33, 1988.
5. Brouns, F., Heat — sweat — dehydration — rehydration: A praxis oriented approach, *J. Sports Sci.*, 9, 143, 1991.
6. Armstrong, L. E., Hubbard, R. W., Jones, B. H., and Daniels, J. T., Preparing Alberto Salazar for the heat of the 1984 olympic marathon, *Phys. Sportsmed.*, 14, 73, 1986.
7. Brouns, F., Saris, W., and Schneider, H., Rationale for upper limits of electrolyte replacement, *Int. J. Sport Nutr.*, 2, 229, 1992.
8. Greenleaf, J. E., and Harrison, M. H., Water and electrolytes, In *Nutrition and Aerobic Exercise*, Layman, D. K., (Ed.), American Chemical Society, Washington, D.C., 1986, 107.
9. Greenleaf, J. E., Problems: thirst, drinking behavior, and involuntary dehydration, *Med. Sci. Sports Exerc.*, 24, 645, 1992.
10. Pivarnik, J. M. and Palmer, R. A., Water and electrolyte balance during rest and exercise, in *Nutrition in Exercise and Sport*, Wolinsky, I., and Hickson, J. F., (Eds.), CRC Press, Inc., Boca Raton, 1994, 245.
11. Sawka, M. N., Young, A. J., Francesconi, R. P., Muza, S. R., and Pandolf, K. B., Thermoregulatory and blood responses during exercise at graded hypohydration levels, *J. Appl. Physiol.*, 59, 1394, 1985.
12. Grandjean, A. C., Hursh, L. M., Majure, W. C., and Hanley, D. F., Nutrition knowledge and practices of college athletes, *Med. Sci. Sports Exerc.*, 13, 82, 1991.
13. Grandjean, A. C., Practices and recommendations of sports nutritionists, *Int. J. Sport Nutr.*, 3, 232, 1993.
14. Rolls, B. J., Palatability and fluid intake, in *Fluid Replacement and Heat Stress*, National Academy Press, Washington, D.C., 1993, 161.
15. Boulze, D., Montastruc, P., and Cabanac, M., Water intake, pleasure and water temperature in humans, *Physiol. Behav.*, 30, 97, 1983.
16. Hubbard, R. W., Sandick, B. L., Matthew, W. T., Francesconi, R. P., Sampson, J. B., Durkot, M. J., Maller, O., and Engell, D. B., Voluntary dehydration and alliesthesia for water, *J. Appl. Physiol.*, 57, 868, 1984.
17. Position of The American Dietetic Association and The Canadian Dietetic Association: Nutrition for physical fitness and athletic peformance for adults, *J. Am. Diet. Assoc.*, 93, 691, 1993.
18. Horswill, C. A., Does rapid weight loss by dehydration adversely affect high-power performance? *Sports Science Exchange*, Gatorade Sports Science Institute, 3, 30, 1991.
19. Steen, S. N. and Brownell, K. D., Patterns of weight loss and regain in wrestlers: has the tradition changed? *Med. Sci. Sports Exerc.*, 22, 762, 1990.

20. Kleiner, S. M., Bazzarre, T. L., and Litchford, M. D., Metabolic profiles, diet, and health practices of championship male and female bodybuilders, *J. Am. Diet. Assoc.,* 90, 962, 1990.

21. Sturmi, J. E. and Rutecki, G. W., When competitive bodybuilders collapse: A result of hyperkalemia? *Phys. Sportsmed.,* 23, 49, 1995.

22. Houston, M. E., Marrin, D. A., Green, H. J., and Thomson, J. A., The effect of rapid weight loss on physiological functions in wrestlers, *Phys. Sportsmed.,* 9, 73, 1981.

23. Burge, C. M., Carey, M. F., and Payne, W. R., Rowing performance, fluid balance, and metabolic function following dehydration and rehydration, *Med. Sci. Sports Exerc.,* 25, 1358, 1993.

24. Gisolfi, C. V. and Duchman, S. M., Guidelines for optimal replacement beverages for different athletic events, *Med. Sci. Sports Exerc.,* 24, 679, 1992.

25. Costill, D. L. and Saltin, B., Factors limiting gastric emptying during rest and exercise, *J. Appl. Physiol.,* 37, 679, 1974.

26. Costill, D. L. and Miller, J. M., Nutrition for endurance sport: carbohydrate and fluid balance, *Int. J. Sports Med.,* 1, 2, 1980.

27. Mitchell, J. B., Costill, D. L., Houmard, J. A., Flynn, M. G., Fink, W. J., and Beltz, J. D., Effects of carbohydrate ingestion on gastric emptying and exercise performance, *Med. Sci. Sports Exerc.,* 20, 110, 1988.

28. Davis, J. M., Lamb, D. R., Pate, R. R., Slentz, C. A., Burgess, W. A., and Bartoli, W. P., Carbohydrate-electrolyte drinks: effects on endurance cycling in the heat, *Am. J. Clin. Nutr.,* 48, 1023, 1988.

29. Mitchell, J. B., Costill, D. L., Houmard, J. A., Fink, W. J., Robergs, R. A., and Davis, J. A., Gastric emptying: influence of prolonged exercise and carbohydrate concentrations, *Med. Sci. Sports Exerc.,* 21, 269, 1989.

30. Murray, R., Paul, G. L., Seifert, J. G., Eddy, D. E., and Halaby, G. A., The effects of glucose, fructose, and sucrose ingestion during exercise, *Med. Sci. Sports Exerc.,* 21, 275, 1989.

31. Below, P. R., Mora-Rodriguez, R., Gonzalez-Alonso, J., and Coyle, E. F., Fluid and carbohydrate ingestion independently improve performance during 1 h of intense exercise, *Med. Sci. Sports Exerc.,* 27, 200, 1995.

32. Coyle, E. F. and Montain, S. J., Benefits of fluid replacement with carbohydrate during exercise. *Med. Sci. Sports Exerc.,* 24, S324, 1992.

33. Tsintzas, O. K., Williams, C., Singh, R., Wilson, W., and Burrin, J., Influence of carbohydrate-electrolyte drinks on marathon running performance, *Eur. J. Appl. Physiol.,* 70, 154, 1995.

34. Millard-Stafford, M., Sparling, P. B., Rosskopf, L. B., Hinson, B. T., and Dicarlo, L. J., Carbohydrate-electrolyte replacement during a simulated triathlon in the heat, *Med. Sci. Sports Exerc.,* 22, 621, 1990.

35. Lyons, T. P., Riedesel, M. L., Meuli, L. E., and Chick, T. W., Effects of glycerol-induced hyperhydration prior to exercise in the heat on sweating and core temperature, *Med. Sci. Sports Exerc.,* 22, 477, 1990.

36. Murray, R., Eddy, D. E., Paul, G. L., Seifert, J. G., and Halaby, G. A., Physiological responses to glycerol ingestion during exercise, *J. Appl. Physiol.,* 71, 144, 1991.

37. Freund, B. J., Montain, S. J., Young, A. J., Sawka, M. N., DeLuca, J. P., Pandolf, K. B., and Valeri, C. R., Glycerol hyperhydration: hormonal, renal, and vascular fluid responses, *J. Appl. Physiol.,* 79, 2069-2077, 1995.

38. Montner, P., Chick, T., Reidesel, M., Timms, M., Stark, D., and Murata, G., Glycerol hyperhydration and endurance exercise, *Med. Sci. Sports Exerc.,* 24, S157, 1992.

39. Armstrong, L. E., Costill, D. L., Fink, W. J., Hargreaves, I., Nishibata, I., Bassett, D., and King, D. S., Effects of dietary sodium intake on body and muscle potassium content in unacclimatized men during successive days of work in the heat, *Eur. J. Appl. Physiol.,* 54, 391, 1985.

40. Nose, H., Mack, G. W., Shi, X., and Nadel, E. R., Role of osmolality and plasma volume during rehydration in humans, *J. Appl. Physiol.*, 65, 325, 1988.
41. Carter, J. E. and Gisolfi, C. V., Fluid replacement during and after exercise in the heat, *Med. Sci. Sports Exerc.*, 21, 532, 1989.
42. Maughan, R. J. and Leiper, J. B., Sodium intake and post-exercise rehydration in man, *Eur. J. Appl. Physiol.*, 71, 311, 1995.
43. Noakes, T. D., The hyponatremia of exercise, *Int. J. Sport Nutr.,* 2, 205, 1992.
44. Frizzell, R. T., Lang, G. H., Lowance, D. C., and Lathan, S. R., Hyponatremia and ultra-marathon running, *J. Am. Med. Assoc.,* 255, 722, 1986.
45. Nelson, P. B., Robinson, A. G., Kapoor, W., and Rinaldo, J., Hyponatremia in a marathoner, *Phys. Sportsmed.*, 16, 78, 1988.
46. Hiller, W. D. B., O'Toole, M. L., and Laird, R. H., Hyponatremia and ultramarathons, *J. Am. Med. Assoc.,* 256, 213, 1986.
47. Haymes, E. M., Vitamin and mineral supplementation to athletes, *Int. J. Sport Nutr.,* 1, 146, 1991.
48. Perez, A., Electrolytes: restoring the balance, *RN*, November, 32, 1995.
49. Food and Nutrition Board, National Research Council, *Recommended Dietary Allowances*, 10th ed., National Academy Press, Washington, D.C., 1989, 256.

Chapter **6**

BODY WEIGHT AND BODY COMPOSITION

CONTENTS

I. INTRODUCTION

Being at the ideal weight or having the ideal body composition is associated with success in many sports. Having too much body fat or too little body fat can result in decreased performance and significant health problems. But what is "ideal" and how is it determined?

Body weight is largely determined by genetics and depends on factors such as body size, body type, and body composition. Body size refers to height and weight, while body type refers to structure and frame. We inherit specific body types or somatotypes. They are

- Ectomorph — lean, slightly muscular
- Mesomorph — naturally muscular and strong, long torso
- Endomorph — stocky build, wide bone structure

Athletes usually have a predominance of one body type with aspects of the other two[1] and are drawn to a particular sport to which they are naturally suited.[2] While athletes cannot change their given body type, they can change their body composition with proper training and nutrition. But first, they need to know more about body composition.

Body composition refers to the chemical make up of the body. Muscle tissue, nerve tissue, bone, ligaments, minerals, and fat are all part of the body's composition. Fat mass is the amount of total body mass that is made up of fat. Fat-free mass consists of lean body mass plus the nonfat components of adipose tissue.[3] The terms fat-free mass and lean body mass are often used interchangeably.

While body size and body type are important factors in determining body weight, body composition is of greater concern. It distinguishes between the overfat vs. the overweight, muscular athlete. Two athletes of equal height and weight can have body compositions that vary significantly.

II. METHODS OF ASSESSING BODY COMPOSITION

Many methods exist to measure lean and fat compartments of the body. They include hydrostatic weighing, skinfold measurements, dual energy X-ray absorptiometry, bioelectrical impedance analysis, total body water, near-infrared interactance, and ultrasound. The accuracy and reliability of any one technique depends on the training and skill of the individual performing the tests and the use of prediction equations specific to the population being assessed.[4] According to Barr et al.,[2] the most reliable, but least valid method of estimating body composition is body weight as determined by height-weight tables, along with calculation of body mass index (BMI). Height-weight tables can be misleading because they do not not account for lean and fat mass; an athlete may be overweight based on height-weight tables, but may be lean as determined by a low body fat percentage.

A. BODY MASS INDEX

Body mass index (BMI), body weight in kilograms divided by height in meters squared, is used as an index of adiposity in the general population. The accepted "good" weight is defined as a BMI between 19 and 25 kg/m^2 for men and women between 19 and 34 years, and 21 to 27 kg/m^2 for those over 35 years.[5] A BMI >30 kg/m^2 is associated with an increased body fat and risk of obesity except in highly muscular athletes.[5] On the other hand, a BMI <19 kg/m^2 may signify excessive leanness and potential eating disorders. According to Bazzarre,[6] BMI is not an ideal measurement for athletes, especially strength-trained athletes, for whom high BMI values would reflect increased lean body mass rather than increased body fat. Pacy et al.[7] also concluded that BMI should not be used to assess body composition in athletes. In their study comparing various methods of body composition assessment, BMI resulted in significantly higher values of percent body fat than any other technique.

B. UNDERWATER WEIGHING

Hydrostatic or underwater weighing has traditionally been viewed as one of the most accurate estimates of body composition, but it is not widely used because equipment is costly and experienced technicians are needed for the analysis. Hydrostatic weighing is based on the principle that fat mass weighs less than fat-free mass. Weight is measured on a scale, and volume is determined by submerging the individual in a tank of water and measuring the amount of water that is displaced. Bone and muscle will sink easily in water, whereas fat tissue floats.

C. SKINFOLD MEASUREMENT

Skinfold measurements and bioelectrical impedance analysis are two simple, inexpensive techniques used to determine body composition. Skinfold procedures involve measuring the thickness of subcutaneous fat tissue at one or more sites on the body. It is one of the least expensive and most versatile methods of estimating percent body fat. Accuracy depends on choosing a prediction equation appropriate for the population for which it is being used, and correctly measuring the same skinfold sites used in the prediction equation.[4] In young adult women, the suprailiac, subscapular, triceps, and thigh skinfolds appear to be particularly important in predicting total body fat.[3]

In a study by Webster and Barr,[8] body fat levels were estimated for female adolescent athletes using six different prediction equations. The authors concluded Jackson and Pollock's[9] quadratic equation for skinfolds, using Lohman's[10] age-adjusted specific constants, were most appropriate for this age group and population.

D. BIOELECTRICAL IMPEDANCE ANALYSIS

Bioelectrical impedance analysis (BIA) is based on the principle that conduction of an applied electrical current is greater in fat-free mass because of higher water and electrolyte content of these tissues relative to fat mass.[11] Electrodes are placed on the wrist and ankle, and a low-level current is passed through the body. The resistance to the flow of electricity is measured and the percentage of body fat is determined by a prediction formula.

Jackson et al.[12] examined the reliability and validity of the BIA method and found it less accurate than either hydrostatic weighing or skinfold measurements. Factors which can influence BIA estimates include hydration level, skin temperature, surface electrolyte content, and blood flow distribution.[11] Caution is indicated when estimating percent body fat values using prediction equations provided by the manufacturers of BIA equipment because these formulas may not be appropriate for athletes.[8] Webster and Barr[8] reported that use of BIA and the manufacturer's prediction equation to calculate percent body fat of young female gymnasts resulted in considerably higher body fat estimates (19.9%) than skinfold measurements (10.3%).

Organ et al.[13] described a new technique for measuring segmental bioelectrical impedance that may resolve some of the limitations associated with current methodology. The impedance index, which measures fat distribution externally at a limited number of sites on the body, may provide direct information on internal fat distribution by electrically sampling the fat content of tissues throughout the body.

III. IDEAL BODY COMPOSITION

Assessing an athlete's body composition can be useful in managing concerns about weight and appearance. Female athletes often have inaccurate perceptions of healthy weight and body fat levels. Knowing what amount of body weight is fat weight and what percentage is lean tissue can help coaches, trainers, and physicians monitor an athlete's nutrition and training program. The ultimate goal is to recommend an optimal weight or body fat level for health and performance, although it is not uncommon for athletes and their coaches to misuse or abuse the information obtained from body composition assessment.[2] Athletes who are told they are too heavy may resort to extreme weight control practices to lose weight.[14]

Many coaches and athletes believe that there are "ideal" body fats for specific sports. However, there is no optimal body fat percentage. Genetics, age, diet, and level of training are factors that influence body fat levels. Athletes should determine their body fat levels based on their performance, not an equivocal number on a chart.[15] Recommendations for percent body fat are usually based on averages obtained from data reported in the literature.[4] As shown in Figure 6.1, there is a wide range of body fat levels among competitive female athletes, ranging from 6 to 20%.

There is also a wide range of body fat levels between athletes within the same sport group. In a study of 15 elite heavyweight women rowers, Pacy et al.[7] reported that percent body fats ranged from 13.6 to 29.3 with a mean of 19.1. Results of this study suggest that setting an "ideal" body fat for an athlete is of limited value.

IV. ENERGY BALANCE

Simply put, body weight is a matter of energy balance — energy intake should equal energy output. Many different factors affect this balance. Hunger, appetite, and satiety influence energy intake while resting metabolic rate, thermic effect of food, and physical activity influence energy expenditure.[16]

Each person has a specific requirement for calories, but the exact number is difficult to determine. Age, sex, body size, and level of activity are important considerations. Generally, an athlete is consuming enough calories if she is maintaining body weight.

The World Health Organization defines energy requirement as "that level of energy intake from food which will balance energy expenditure when the individual has a body size and composition, and level of physical activity, consistent with long-term health; and which will allow for the maintenance of economically necessary and socially desirable physical activity."[17]

Recommended energy intakes published by the National Research Council appear in Table 6.1.[18] These energy values are based on individuals with light-to-moderate activity level. The average daily energy intake for the referenced 19- to 24-year-old female is 2200 kcal or 38 kcal/kg. Many sedentary women require less energy than standard weight tables suggest. On the other hand, the serious competitive athlete may need 700 to 1000 additional calories to support her training and competitive schedule.

Several different formulas have been developed for estimating energy expenditure, some of which are quite complicated. A simple way to determine calorie need is to multiply weight in pounds by using one of the numbers provided in Table 6.2. For example, a 64 kg (140 lb) female athlete with a moderate activity level would require approximately 2240 kcal (16 x 140 = 2240).

A. MEASURING ENERGY INTAKE

Energy intake can be estimated by several different methods including 24-hour dietary recall, diet history, food frequency questionnaire, food record, and weighed food intake. Most of these methods have some degree of validity.[19] The method of choice depends on the purpose of the assessment, the sample size, and availability of personnel.[20] The 24-hour recall and food record are the tools most often used to assess energy intakes of athletes. Although the 24-hour recall is reliable for measuring group means, it is not practical for

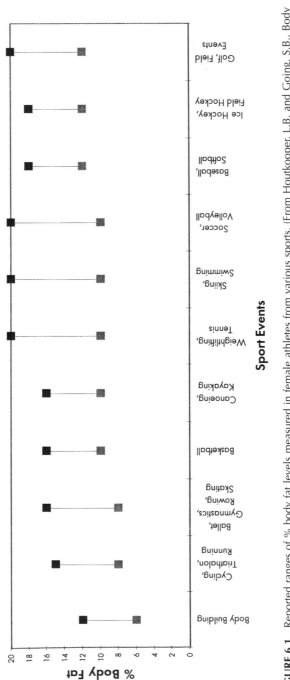

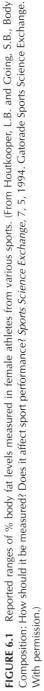

FIGURE 6.1 Reported ranges of % body fat levels measured in female athletes from various sports. (From Houtkooper, L.B. and Going, S.B., Body Composition: How should it be measured? Does it affect sport performance? *Sports Science Exchange, 7*, 5, 1994. Gatorade Sports Science Exchange. With permission.)

TABLE 6.1 Median Heights and Weights and Recommended Energy Intakes (For Females)

	Children	Females						Pregnant	Lactating
Age (Years)	7–10	11–14	15–18	19–24	5–50	51+		Second and Third Trimesters	
Weight									
(kg)	28	46	55	58	63	65			
(lb)	62	101	120	128	138	143			
Height									
(cm)	132	157	163	164	163	160			
(in)	52	62	64	65	64	63			
Average Energy Allowance									
REE (kcal/d)	1130	1310	1370	1350	1380	1280			
Multiples of REE		1.67	1.60	1.60	1.55	1.50			
Kcal/kg	70	47	40	38	36	30			
Kcal/d	2000	2200	2200	2200	2200	1900		+300	+500

Adapted from the Food and Nutrition Board, National Research Council, *Recommended Dietary Allowances*, 10th ed., National Academy Press, Washington, D.C., 1989.

TABLE 6.2	Factors for Estimating Daily Energy Allowances at Various Levels of Physical Activity for Women Ages 19 to 50[a]

Activity Level	Activity Factor
Light	13
Moderate	16
Heavy	19
Exceptional	22

[a] Adapted from the Food and Nutrition Board, *Recommended Dietary Allowances,* National Research Council, 10th ed., National Academy Press, Washington, D.C., 1989.

assessing the usual diet of individuals. The number of days for which food records are obtained affects the usefulness of the data. In a nationwide survey of the nutritional habits of elite athletes, van Erp-Baart et al.[21] found that recording for 4 days including the weekend gives better information than a 24-hour recall.

Several studies have reported discrepancies between reported energy intake and energy expenditure suggesting that individuals may underestimate food intake.[22-24] de Vries et al.[23] calculated self-reported energy intakes from 3-day dietary records with actual intakes needed to maintain body weight and found that subjects underestimated their energy intake by 10%. Mertz et al.[22] also found underreporting to be common among the general population: 81% of the subjects reported their energy intake at approximately 700 kcal below the amount required to maintain body weight.

Investigators have also noted changes in energy and nutrient intakes during the menstrual cycle.[25-27] In a study by Martini et al.,[27] 3-day diet records were collected 6 to 8 days after menstruation and 6 to 8 days after ovulation. Mean energy intake was significantly higher during the luteal phase than during the follicular phase, 1908 kcal/d and 1749 kcal/d, respectively. Higher intakes of protein, carbohydrates, and fat were also reported. These results are consistent with those of Tarasuk and Beaton[26] who also reported higher energy and fat intakes during the luteal phase of the menstrual cycle.

B. FACTORS INFLUENCING ENERGY EXPENDITURE

The body uses energy in three ways, through basal metabolic rate, also referred to as resting metabolic rate, physical activity, and the thermic effect of food. An explanation of these follows.

1. Basal Metabolic Rate

Basal metabolism is the energy level required to maintain life-sustaining activities like breathing, circulation, and heart beat. It is measured in terms of basal metabolic rate (BMR), the rate at which the body uses energy to keep all these life-supporting processes going.

Basal metabolic rate is the largest contributor to total energy expenditure, accounting for 60 to 70% of daily energy needs.[16] A female may expend as many as 1,067 to 2,853 kcal/d to support basal metabolism.[28]

Basal metabolic rate is affected by several factors:

- Age. A person's BMR is greatest during infancy.
- Fat-free mass. This accounts for the greatest source of variation in BMR in humans.[29] The more lean tissue the higher the BMR; the more fat tissue, the lower the BMR.
- Gender. BMR is about 3% lower in women than in men, independent of body composition and activity level.[30]
- Body temperature. Fever significantly increases BMR. A cold external temperature also raises BMR as the body attempts to stay warm.
- Physiological status. The thyroid hormone, thyroxine, is a key regulator of BMR. The more thyroxine produced, the higher is the BMR. Conditions such as pregnancy, menstruation, and eating disorder practices influence BMR.

2. Physical Activity

Physical activity is the second largest influence on energy expenditure. It constitutes 15 to 30% of total energy needs.[16] The amount of energy used by an athlete depends on the type of sport, physical conditioning, clothing worn, playing surface, and frequency, intensity, and duration of the event or training session. Among well-trained female athletes, energy expended in physical activity can be as high as 36 to 38% of daily energy expenditure.[31,32] Body size impacts energy expenditure more than any other single factor. Tall athletes with a large lean body mass use more energy to perform a given task than do smaller, less muscular athletes.

3. Thermic Effect of Food

The third component of energy expenditure is the energy required for the body to digest, absorb, metabolize, and store food. When food is consumed, the activity in the cells increases. This increase in cellular activity is known as the thermic effect of food (TEF) or diet-induced thermogenesis. The thermic effect is relatively small, accounting for about 7 to 10% of total energy needs, or about 120 to 170 kcal/d for women.[33] Some data have shown that female athletes have a lower TEF, indicating that they may be more energy efficient than nonathletes.[34] However, other studies have found no differences.[35-37]

C. MEASURING ENERGY EXPENDITURE

Energy expenditure can be measured by a number of methods including direct calorimetry, indirect calorimetry, and noncalorimetric methods. Although both direct and indirect calorimetry yield excellent accuracy in laboratory settings, the relevance for athletes under normal training situations is questionable.[38] In 1982, the doubly-labeled water technique, a noncalorimetric method of estimating energy expenditure, was first used by Schoeller and van Santen[39] in human subjects. Doubly-labeled water is a method of measuring carbon dioxide, which is the end product of the oxidation of food. This procedure has been validated for estimating energy expenditure. In female athletes, comparisons between reported energy intake and energy expenditure have been made using the doubly-labeled water technique.[24,32,38] Edwards et al.[24] reported a 32% difference in the mean daily values for energy expenditure compared to energy intake in highly trained female runners. However, no change in body weight occurred. The authors concluded that female athletes underreported food intake.

1. Energy Balance in Female Athletes

Studies determining energy balance in female athletes have consistently found discrepancies between reported energy intake and energy expenditure.[24,35,40-43] Researchers have questioned why some female athletes are not losing weight if reported energy intakes indeed reflect day to day eating habits.[43,44] One explanation may be the decrease in resting metabolic rate that reportedly occurs in response to calorie restriction.[45] Other possible factors include errors in methods used to determine energy intake and/or expenditure,[44] underreporting of food intake,[24] or restricted eating during the measurement period.[22,24,35,37] Inaccuracies in the nutrient database are also possible.

Some investigators say that highly trained female athletes are able to maintain body weight without an appreciable increase in energy intake.[46,47] However, Horton et al.[31] found no significant increase in energy efficiency of female cyclists compared to a control group. They measured usual energy intake from self-selected diets, and determined energy expenditure using indirect calorimetry. Athletes maintained energy balance by consuming more calories on cycling days compared with noncycling days.

V. ACHIEVING A HEALTHY COMPETITIVE WEIGHT

Helping the female athlete achieve a healthy competitive weight is important for many reasons. Psychologically, the athlete who feels good about her body weight and appearance has better eating habits and food-related behaviors than one who does not. Dissatisfaction with body weight leads to dieting which can contribute to weight cycling (repeated weight loss and weight gain), eating disorders, menstrual dysfunction, and bone mineral disorders in female athletes.

Physiologically, maintaining an optimal body weight has important health and performance implications. Being overweight (20% increase in body weight) is associated with increased risk for coronary heart disease, diabetes, and some forms of cancer in women.[48] Experience shows that athletes who achieve and maintain an optimal body weight throughout training and competition generally exhibit better overall performance.

Storlie[49] recommends a three-step process for determining an athlete's optimal body weight. The first step is to obtain the athlete's personal weight goal. How much does she want to weigh? Is her weight goal realistic? The next step is to assess body composition to determine a desirable body weight range. Anthropometric measurements such as height/weight and skinfolds are practical and cost-effective methods for estimating body composition, although the limitations of these techniques should be recognized. The final step in determining ideal body weight is to identify a realistic target weight based on age and performance goals.

A. WEIGHT LOSS PLAN

The goal of a weight loss plan should be to decrease body fat while maintaining lean body mass. This can be accomplished through a balanced diet, exercise, and behavior modification.

1. A Balanced Diet

The most successful approach to weight loss, as well as weight maintenance is a safe, nutritious diet that complements individual food tastes and lifestyles. Athletes who give up foods they enjoy will find it much harder to achieve their weight goals. A sound weight loss plan should include foods from the five major food groups, with special emphasis on nutrient-dense foods (Figure 6.2) Diets that rely on special food products or eliminate one or more food groups will not provide the proper nutrients and will not help the athlete learn a better way of eating.

A gradual weight loss is recommended and can be achieved by decreasing calories and increasing energy expenditure. One lb (0.5 kg) of body fat is equal to about 3500 kcal. To lose 0.5 to 0.9 kg (1 to 2 lb) per week, the athlete will need to reduce calorie intake by 500 to 1000 kcal/d. Starvation or very-low-calorie diets are not ever recommended, because of the possible detrimental effects on health and performance. Very restrictive diets can result in nutrition deficiencies, dehydration, glycogen depletion, loss of lean body mass, electrolyte imbalances, and increased risk of illness and injury.

When total caloric intake is less than 1200 kcal/d, it becomes increasingly difficult to get the recommended amounts of essential nutrients. As previously stated, female athletes who limit calories, frequently consume less than 75% of the RDA for many vitamins and minerals. However, one should not assume that adequate calorie intake ensures good nutrition. In a study of triathletes, Green et al.[50] reported that female triathletes consuming an average of 4,149 kcal/d had low intakes of several vitamins and minerals. Green et al.[50] concluded that training and work schedules hampered appropriate food choices. The athletes selected mostly high-calorie, low nutrient-dense foods.

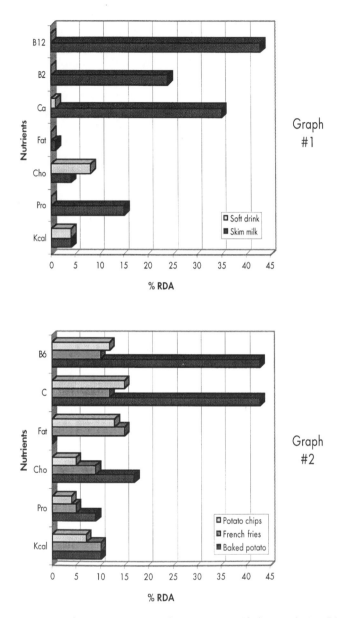

FIGURE 6.2 Nutrient density, a measure of nutrients provided per calorie of food, is a valuable concept used in diet planning. The idea is to maximize nutrients and minimize calories; a more nutrient-dense food has fewer calories and usually less fat. The graphs above show the nutrient density of two different food items. Compare the nutritional composition of a baked potato (with no fat), french fries and potato chips. All three foods provide vitamin C, but the potato is "denser" in vitamin C. Likewise, skim milk is denser in calcium than a soft drink. (From Nutrition for Women, Part II, Dale Ames Kline, Nutrition Dimension, Inc., 1991.)

The best dietary advice for weight loss is to consume a low-fat, high-carbohydrate diet with an increased fiber content.[51] As recommended in the dietary guidelines, fat intake should contribute no more than 30% of total calories in the diet. Many female athletes have become preoccupied with eating low-fat foods in an effort to lose weight. However, recent data show that in some cases, the emphasis on low-fat foods may actually contribute to weight gain. According to Allred,[52] "many individuals believe that if a food is low in fat, they can have as many servings as they want without gaining weight." A low-fat food is not always low in calories. Health professionals working with athletes need to reemphasize total calorie intake as well as portion control.

2. The Role of Exercise

Regular exercise plays an important role in both the prevention and treatment of obesity. Research shows that calorie restriction alone is not as effective as calorie restriction combined with exercise. Mole et al.[53] demonstrated that dieting with exercise stimulated energy expenditure and fat oxidation, leading to a reduction in body fat. In another study, Hill et al.[54] reported that moderate exercise in conjunction with a high-carbohydrate, moderate protein, low-fat diet led to a greater total weight loss and a greater decrease in percent body fat. The study also suggested that subjects who exercise during and after weight loss are better able to maintain body weight than those who do not exercise. However, increased aerobic activity may not be practical for the athlete who already trains several hours a day. Changing the type of exercise may promote changes in body composition. Recent data by Wilmore[55] observed greater decreases in fat mass in weight training compared to aerobic training. More research is needed to confirm this observation.

B. BEHAVIOR MODIFICATION

To lose weight safely and keep it off, a permanent change in eating behaviors must occur. Many female athletes have developed eating patterns that make weight control difficult. Behavior modification is a formal process that can help individuals make changes in eating behaviors. Behavior modification involves four basic steps:[56]

- Identifying eating or related lifestyle behaviors to be modified
- Setting specific behavior goals
- Modifying elements of the behavior to be changed
- Reinforcing the desired behavior

The first step is usually an analysis of the athlete's eating behavior. The athlete is instructed to keep a careful record containing such information as daily food intake and factors associated with eating, such as where and when eating occurs, who is present, degree of hunger, and emotions. This record is used to determine what conditions can lead to good eating habits.

After an initial assessment, therapy is directed toward specific aspects of eating behavior. One technique might be a more controlled rate of eating. For example, the athlete might be taught to eat at a slower pace and leave some food on the plate. Another recommendation is to learn appropriate portion sizes. The ultimate goal is to modify eating and physical activity habits, focusing on gradual changes.

VI. CONCLUSIONS

Body weight is largely determined by genetics and depends on an athlete's body size, body type, and body composition. Many methods are available to assess body composition. The most practical and inexpensive methods include anthropometric measurements such as height/weight and skinfold measurements. There is no ideal body fat level for specific sports. Athletes should determine their body fat levels based on their performance. Nevertheless, many female athletes strive for extremely low body fat levels that can result in decreased performance and significant health problems.

To maintain body weight, energy intake should balance energy expenditure. Many different factors affect this balance and have been discussed in this chapter. Some experts believe that female athletes underreport energy intakes which may reflect concerns about weight and body image.

REFERENCES

1. Wilmore, J. and Costill, D., *Physiology of Sport and Exercise,* Human Kinetics, Champaign, Il, 1994, 382.
2. Barr, S. I., McCargar, L. J., and Crawford, S. M., Practical use of body composition analysis in sport, *Sports Med.*, 17, 277, 1994.
3. Jensen, M. D., Research techniques for body composition assessment, *J. Am. Diet. Assoc.*, 92, 454, 1992.
4. Houtkooper, L. B. and Going, S. B., Body composition: How should it be measured? Does it affect sport performance?, *Sports Science Exchange*, Gatorade Sports Science Institute, 7, 5, 1994.
5. Bray, G. A., Pathophysiology of obesity, *Am. J. Clin. Nutr.*, 55, 488S, 1992.
6. Bazzarre, T. L., Nutrition and Strength, In *Nutrition in Exercise and Sport*, Wolinsky, I. and Hickson, J. F., Eds., CRC Press, Inc., Boca Raton, 1994, 418.
7. Pacy, P. J., Quevedo, M., Gibson, N. R., Cox, M., Koutedakis, Y., and Millward, J., Body composition measurement in elite heavyweight oarswomen: a comparison of five methods, *J. Sports Med. Phys. Fitness*, 35, 67, 1995.
8. Webster, B. L. and Barr, S. I., Body composition analysis of female adolescent athletes: comparing six regression equations, *Med. Sci. Sports Exerc.*, 25, 648, 1993.
9. Jackson, A. S., Pollock, M. L., and Ward, A., Generalized equations for predicting body density of women, *Med. Sci. Sports Exerc.*, 12, 175, 1980.
10. Lohman, T. G., Applicability of body composition techniques and constants for children and youths, *Exerc. Sport Sci. Rev.*, 14, 325, 1984.

11. Lukaski, H. C., Bolonchuk, W. W., Siders, W. A., and Hall, C. B., Body composition assessment of athletes using bioelectrical impedance measurements, *J. Sports Med. Phys. Fitness*, 30, 434, 1990.

12. Jackson, A. S., Pollock, M. I., Graves, J. E., and Mahar, M. T., Reliability and validity of bioelectrical impedance in determining body composition, *J. Appl. Physiol.*, 64, 529, 1988.

13. Organ, L. W., Bradham, G. B., Gore, D. T., and Lozier, S. L., Segmental bioelectrical impedance analysis: theory and application of a new technique, *J. Appl. Physiol.*, 77, 98, 1994.

14. Rosen, L. W. and Hough, D. O., Pathogenic weight-control behaviors of female college gymnasts, *Phys. Sportsmed.*, 16, 141, 1988.

15. Oppliger, R. A. and Cassady, S. L., Body composition assessment in women: special considerations for athletes, *Sports Med.*, 17, 353, 1994.

16. Poehlman, E. T., A review: exercise and its influence on resting energy metabolism in man, *Med. Sci. Sports Exerc.*, 21, 515, 1989.

17. World Health Organization, *Energy and protein requirements*, Report of Joint FAO/WHO/UNU Expert Consultation, Technical Report Series 724, Geneva, World Health Organization, 1985.

18. Food and Nutrition Board, National Research Council, *Recommended Dietary Allowances*, 10th ed., National Academy Press, Washington, D.C., 1989, 29.

19. Block, G., A review of validations of dietary assessment methods, *Am. J. Epidemiol.*, 115, 492, 1982.

20. Pekkarinen, M., Methodology in the collection of food consumption data, In *World Review of Nutrition and Dietetics*, Bourne, G. H., Ed., Basel S. Karger, 12, 145, 1970.

21. van Erp-Baart, A. M. J., Saris, W. H. M., Binkhorst, R. A., Vos, J. A., and Elvers, J. W. H., Nationwide survey on nutritional habits in elite athletes, *Int. J. Sports Med.*, 10, S3, 1989.

22. Mertz, W., Tsui, J. C., Judd, J. T., Reiser, S., Hallfrisch, J., Morris, E. R., Steele, P. D., and Lashley, E., What are people really eating? The relation between energy intake derived from estimated diet records and intake determined to maintain body weight, *Am. J. Clin. Nutr.*, 54, 291, 1991.

23. de Vries, J. H. M., Zock, P. L., Mensink, R. P., and Katan, M. B., Underestimation of energy intake by 3-d records compared with energy intake to maintain body weight in 269 nonobese adults, *Am. J. Clin. Nutr.*, 60, 855, 1994.

24. Edwards, J. E., Lindeman, A. K., Mikesky, A. E., and Stager, J. M., Energy balance in highly trained female endurance runners, *Med. Sci. Sports Exerc.*, 25, 1398, 1993.

25. Gong, E. J., Garrel, D., and Calloway, D. H., Menstrual cycle and voluntary food intake, *Am. J. Clin. Nutr.*, 49, 252, 1989.

26. Tarasuk, V. and Beaton, G. H., Menstrual-cycle patterns in energy and macronutrient intake, *Am. J. Clin. Nutr.*, 53, 442, 1991.

27. Martini, M. C., Lampe, J. W., Slavin, J. L., and Kurzer, M. S., Effect of the menstrual cycle on energy and nutrient intake, *Am. J. Clin. Nutr.*, 60, 895, 1994.

28. Tataranni, P. A. and Ravussin, E., Variability in metabolic rate: biological sites of regulation, *Int. J. Obesity*, 19, S102, 1995.

29. Poehlman, E. T., Berke, E. M., Joseph, J. R., Gardner, A. W., Katzman-Rooks, S. M., and Goran, M. I., Influence of aerobic capacity, body composition, and thyroid hormones on the age-related decline in resting metabolic rate, *Metabolism*, 41, 915, 1992.

30. Arciero, P. J., Goran, M. I., and Poehlman, E. T., Resting metabolic rate is lower in women than in men, *J. Appl. Physiol.*, 75, 2514, 1993.

31. Horton, T. J., Drougas, H. J., Sharp, T. A., Martinez, L. R., Reed, G. W., and Hill, J. O., Energy balance in endurance-trained female cyclists and untrained controls, *J. Appl. Physiol.*, 76, 1937, 1994.

32. Schulz, L. O., Alger, S., Harper, I., Wilmore, J. H., and Ravussin, E., Energy expenditure of elite female runners measured by respiratory chamber and doubly labeled water, *J. Appl. Physiol.*, 72, 23, 1992.

33. Ravussin, E., Lillioja, S., Anderson, T. E., Christin, L., and Bogardus, C., Determinants of 24-hour energy expenditure in man, *J. Clin. Invest.*, 78, 1568, 1986.
34. LeBlanc, J., Diamond, P., Cote, J., and Labrie, A., Hormonal factors in reduced postprandial heat production of exercise-trained subjects, *J. Appl. Physiol.*, 56, 772, 1984.
35. Beidleman, B. A., Puhl, J. L., and De Souza, J., Energy balance in female distance runners, *Am. J. Clin. Nutr.*, 61, 303, 1995.
36. Myerson, M., Gutin, B., Warren, M. P., May, M. T., Contento, I., Lee, M., Pi-Sunyer, F. X., Pierson, R. N., and Brooks-Gunn, J., Resting metabolic rate and energy balance in amenorrheic and eumenorrheic runners, *Med. Sci. Sports Exerc.*, 23, 15, 1991.
37. Wilmore, J. H., Wambsgans, K. C., Brenner, M., Broeder, C. E., Paijmans, I., Volpe, J. A., and Wilmore, K. M., Is there energy conservation in amenorrheic compared with eumenorrheic distance runners? *J. Appl. Physiol.*, 72, 15, 1992.
38. Sjodin, A. M., Andersson, A. B., Hogberg, J. M., and Westerterp, K. R., Energy balance in cross-country skiers: a study using doubly labeled water, *Med. Sci. Sport Exerc.*, 26, 720, 1994.
39. Schoeller, D. A. and van Santen, E., Measurement of energy expenditure in humans by doubly labeled water method, *J. Appl. Physiol.*, 53, 955, 1982.
40. Deuster, P. A., Kyle, S. B., Moser, P. B., Vigersky, R. A., Singh, A., and Schoomaker, E. B., Nutritional survey of highly trained women runners, *Am. J. Clin. Nutr.*, 44, 954, 1986.
41. Pate, R. R., Sargent, R. G., Baldwin, C., and Burgess, M. L., Dietary intake of woman runners, *Int. J. Sports Med.*, 11, 461, 1990.
42. Keith, R. E., O'Keeffe, K. A., Alt, L. A., and Young, K. L., Dietary status of trained female cyclists, *J. Am. Diet. Assoc.*, 89, 1620, 1989.
43. Barr, S. I., Women, nutrition and exercise: a review of athletes' intakes and a discussion of energy balance in active women, *Prog. Food and Nutr. Sci.*, 11, 307, 1987.
44. Dahlstrom, M., Jansson, E., Nordevang, E., and Kaijser, L., Discrepancy between estimated energy intake and requirement in female dancers, *Clin. Physiol.*, 10, 11, 1990.
45. Henson, L. C., Poole, D. C., Donahoe, C. P., and Heber, D., Effects of exercise training on resting energy expenditure during caloric restriction, *Am. J. Clin. Nutr.*, 46, 893, 1987.
46. Mulligan, K. and Butterfield, G. E., Discrepancies between energy intake and expenditure in physically active women, *Br. J. Nutr.*, 64, 23, 1990.
47. Vallieres, F., Tremblay, A., and St-Jean, L., Study of the energy balance and the nutritional status of highly trained female swimmers, *Nutr. Res.*, 9, 699, 1989.
48. St. Joer, S. T., The role of weight management in the health of women, *J. Am. Diet. Assoc.*, 93, 1007, 1993.
49. Storlie, J., Nutrition assessment of athletes: A model for integrating nutrition and physical performance indicators, *Int. J. Sport Nutr.*, 1, 192, 1991.
50. Green, D. R., Gibbons, C., O'Toole, M., and Hiller, W. B. O., An evaluation of dietary intakes of triathletes: Are RDAs being met? *J. Am. Diet. Assoc.*, 89, 1653, 1989.
51. Rolls, B. J., Carbohydrates, fats, and satiety, *Am. J. Clin. Nutr.*, 61, 960S, 1995.
52. Allred, J. B., Too much of a good thing? *J. Am. Diet. Assoc.*, 95, 417, 1995.
53. Mole, P. A., Stern, J. S., Schultz, C. L., Bernauer, E. M., and Holcomb, B. J., Exercise reverses depressed metabolic rate produced by severe caloric restriction, *Med. Sci. Sports Exerc.*, 21, 29, 1989.
54. Hill, J. O., Schlundt, D. G., Sbrocco, T., Sharp, T., Pope-Cordle, J., Stetson, B., Kaler, M., and Heim, C., Evaluation of an alternating-calorie diet with and without exercise in the treatment of obesity, *Am. J. Clin. Nutr.*, 50, 248, 1989.
55. Wilmore, J. H., Variations in physical activity habits and body composition, *Int. J. Obesity*, 19, S107, 1995.
56. NIH Technology Assessment Conference Panel, Methods for voluntary weight loss and control. *Ann. Intern. Med.*, 116, 942, 1992.

Chapter 7

EATING DISORDERS IN ATHLETES

CONTENTS

I. INTRODUCTION

In her book, *Reviving Ophelia*, Mary Pipher, a clinical psychologist, encourages health professionals, parents, and educators to "build a culture that is less complicated and more nurturing" for adolescent girls.[1] The theme of the book, saving the selves of adolescent girls, is based on the story of Ophelia, from Shakespeare's *Hamlet*.

Throughout the book, Pipher illustrates the enormous pressure young girls feel to be attractive and achieve a certain body weight. She attributes this preoccupation with weight to American cultural values and to the media's presentation of women.

This worship of the perfect body can have serious psychological and behavioral consequences. As girls grow older and their bodies change, they become increasingly dissatisfied with some aspect of their appearance.[2] In a survey of 854 adolescent girls and young women, Moore[3] reported that 67% were dissatisfied with weight, and 54% were dissatisfied with body shape. Of those who viewed themselves as overweight 36% desired an inappropriate weight loss.

Concerns about body weight and body dissatisfaction are also prevalent among female athletes.[4-9] This is especially true for athletes who must maintain a low body weight or low body fat for their sport. Davis and Cowles[9] reported that athletes in "thin-build" sports (gymnastics, figure skating, long distance running, ballet) had greater weight concerns, more body dissatisfaction and more persistent dieting than athletes in normal build sports (field hockey, basketball, sprinting, volleyball).

The inability to control weight and body shape can lead to a multitude of nutrition-related health problems, the most severe of which are anorexia nervosa and bulimia nervosa. Restrictive dieting can lead to nutritional inadequacies, amenorrhea, iron deficiency, and low bone mineral density. Dehydration is also common in athletes who diet excessively, binge and purge, or use diuretics and laxatives.

Coaches, team physicians, and sports nutritionists need to be aware of athletes with weight concerns and help them achieve a body weight that promotes optimal health and performance. This chapter presents an overview of eating disorders in athletes, including definition and diagnostic criteria, prevalence, risk factors, and effects on health and performance.

II. DEFINITION AND DIAGNOSTIC CRITERIA

According to the revised fourth edition of *The Diagnostic and Statistical Manual of Mental Disorders (DSM-IV)*,[10] eating disorders are characterized by severe disturbances in eating behavior. The term eating disorder typically refers to anorexia nervosa or bulimia nervosa. However, eating disorder has recently been applied to eating disorders not otherwise specified (NOS), such as anorexia athletica and binge-eating disorder, categories for disorders of eating that do not meet the criteria for anorexia or bulimia.

Up to 0.5 to 1% of adolescent and young adult women have anorexia nervosa, and 1 to 3% have bulimia nervosa.[10] Many cases go unnoticed. Coaches, trainers, team physicians, and sports nutritionists need to be aware of the early signs of eating disorders so that preventive steps can be taken.

A. ANOREXIA NERVOSA

Anorexia nervosa is characterized in individuals by a refusal to maintain body weight over a minimally normal weight for age and height, an intense fear of gaining weight or becoming fat, a distorted body image, and in postmenarcheal

TABLE 7.1   Diagnostic Criteria for Anorexia Nervosa

1. Refusal to maintain body weight at or above a minimally normal weight for age and height (e.g., weight loss leading to maintenance of body weight less than 85% of that expected; or failure to make expected weight gain during period of growth, leading to body weight less than 85% of that expected).
2. Intense fear of gaining weight or becoming fat, even though underweight.
3. Disturbance in the way in which one's body weight or shape is experienced, undue influence of body weight or shape on self-evaluation, or denial of the seriousness of the current low body weight.
4. In postmenarcheal females, amenorrhea, i.e., the absence of at least three consecutive menstrual cycles. (A woman is considered to have amenorrhea if her periods occur only following hormone, e.g., estrogen, administration.)

Specify type:

Restricting Type: during the current episode of Anorexia Nervosa, the person has not regularly engaged in binge-eating or purging behavior (i.e., self-induced vomiting or the misuse of laxatives, diuretics, or enemas)
Binge-Eating/Purging Type: during the current episode of Anorexia Nervosa, the person has regularly engaged in binge-eating or purging behavior (i.e., self-induced vomiting or the misuse of laxatives, diuretics, or enemas)

From American Psychiatric Association: *Diagnostic and Statistical Manual of Mental Disorders,* Fourth Edition, Washington, D.C., American Psychiatric Association, 1994. With permission.

females, amenorrhea, i.e., the absence of at least three consecutive menstrual cycles[10] (Table 7.1).

Anorexics often appear malnourished due to extreme thinness. Yet, when looking in a mirror, they envision themselves as fat. A typical behavior in anorexia is a constant preoccupation with food, dieting, and weight. Issues related to weight or food become highly emotional.

Anorexia is a potentially life-threatening disorder. Although many young women undergo a single episode of anorexia nervosa and fully recover, if unnoticed, anorexia nervosa results in a mortality rate of over 10% from starvation, suicide, or electrolyte imbalance.[11] The death of gymnast and Olympic hopeful Christy Heinrich in 1994 increased awareness of anorexia nervosa and how it can totally consume the life of an athlete.[12] Fortunately, most athletes do not reach extreme levels of eating disorders. Instead, they exhibit less severe or subclinical forms of eating disorders.[13]

It is estimated that in the general population 0.5 to 1% of adolescents and young adult females suffer from anorexia.[10] The prevalence of anorexia nervosa in males is not known.

B. BULIMIA NERVOSA

Bulimia nervosa is described as recurring episodes of binge eating, usually followed by purging (Table 7.2). Vomiting, laxative abuse, and intense exercise are methods used to relieve guilt and prevent weight gain. To qualify for the

TABLE 7.2   Diagnostic Criteria for Bulimia Nervosa

1. Recurrent episodes of binge eating. An episode of binge eating is characterized
   by both of the following:
   a. eating in a discrete period of time (e.g., within any 2-hour period), an amount
      of food that is definitely larger than most people would eat during a similar
      period of time and under similar circumstances
   b. a sense of lack of control over eating during the episode (e.g., a feeling that
      one cannot stop eating or control what or how much one is eating)
2. Recurrent inappropriate compensatory behavior in order to prevent weight gain,
   such as self-induced vomiting; misuse of laxatives, diuretics, enemas, or other
   medications; fasting; or excessive exercise.
3. The binge eating and inappropriate compensatory behaviors both occur, on
   average, at least twice a week for 3 months.
4. Self-evaluation is unduly influenced by body shape and weight.
5. The disturbance does not occur exclusively during episodes of Anorexia Nervosa.

Specify type:

Purging Type: during the current episode of Bulimia Nervosa, the person has regularly
   engaged in self-induced vomiting or the misuse of laxatives, diuretics, or enemas
Nonpurging Type: during the current episode of Bulimia Nervosa, the person has
   used other inappropriate compensatory behaviors, such as fasting or excessive
   exercise, but has not regularly engaged in self-induced vomiting or the misuse of
   laxatives, diuretics, or enemas

From American Psychiatric Association: *Diagnostic and Statistical Manual of Mental
Disorders,* Fourth Edition, Washington, D.C., American Psychiatric Association, 1994.
With permission.

diagnosis, the binge eating and purging must occur, on average, at least twice
a week for three months.[10]

Individuals with bulimia often consume a normal diet but binge to cope
with or avoid emotional stress. Binge eating usually occurs in an attempt to
control weight and feelings about body image. Bulimics, by their very nature,
are secretive and inconspicuous which is why this disorder is often difficult
to diagnose.

Unlike anorexia nervosa, many physical signs of bulimia such as swollen
parotid glands, dental and gum disease, and menstrual irregularities, do not
appear until late in the course of the illness. Additionally, individuals with
bulimia usually appear within the normal weight range, although some may
be slightly underweight or overweight.[10] The incidence of bulimia nervosa is
estimated at 1 to 3% of the adolescent and young adult female population.[10]

C. ANOREXIA ATHLETICA

Sundgot-Borgen[14] has further described a subclinical eating disorder
known as anorexia athletica. The diagnostic criteria for anorexia athletica are
presented in Table 7.3. These features originally were developed by Pulgiese

TABLE 7.3   Diagnostic Criteria for Anorexia Athletica

Weight loss (<5% of expected bodyweight)	+
Delayed puberty [no menstrual bleeding at age 16 (primary amenorrhea)]	(+)
Menstrual dysfunction (primary amenorrhea, secondary amenorrhea and oligomenorrhea)	(+)
Gastrointestinal complaints	(+)
Absence of medical illness or affective disorder explaining the weight reduction	+
Distorted body image	(+)
Excessive fear of becoming obese	+
Restriction of food (<1200 kcal/day)	+
Use of purging methods (self-induced vomiting, use of laxatives and diuretics)	(+)
Binge eating	(+)
Compulsive exercise	(+)

Symbols: + denotes absolute criteria; (+) denotes relative criteria.

From Sundgot-Borgen, J. Eating disorders in female athletes, *Sports Med.,* 17, 176, 1994. With permission.

et al.[15] in 1983 and later modified by Sundgot-Borgen.[14] Distinguishing features of anorexia athletica include (1) an intense fear of gaining weight or becoming fat even though an individual is already underweight (at least 5% less than expected normal weight for age and height for the general female population), (2) restriction of food (<1200 kcal/d), and, (3) compulsive exercise.

Smith[16] was among the first to alert the medical community to the problem of excessive weight loss and food aversion in athletes. According to Smith,[16] the athlete is abnormally preoccupied with food and experiences extreme weight loss, but does not suffer from severe, underlying emotional problems.

III. PREVALENCE OF EATING DISORDERS IN ATHLETES

Data on the prevalence of eating disorders in athletes varies with the diagnostic tool used to measure eating disorders and with the sport.[17] Most of the studies examining the prevalence of eating disorders have used the Eating Attitudes Test (EAT) and the Eating Disorder Inventory (EDI). The EAT is a 40-item measure of eating and dieting behaviors and attitudes associated with eating disorders.[18] A cutoff score of 30 is used to classify individuals who have eating disorders. The EDI is a 64-item, multiscale measure designed to assess a wide range of psychological and behavioral traits common in individuals with eating disorders.[19]

Both the EAT and EDI are standardized self-report instruments with demonstrated reliability and validity. However, one must use caution when making conclusions about the prevalence of eating disorders based on the use of these instruments alone.[13] The EAT and EDI were developed for use in nonclinical settings to assess attitudes and behaviors of individuals consistent with those exhibited by persons with eating disorders.[18,19]

Sundgot-Borgen[17] used the EDI and a self-developed questionnaire to identify individuals at risk for eating disorders. She found that athletes under-reported use of purging methods such as laxatives, diuretics, and vomiting and over-reported binging behaviors. Reasons why athletes may not accurately report weight control behaviors and attitudes include fear of being discovered by coaches, trainers, or teammates, and/or fear of losing their position on the team.[17]

Although the prevalence of eating disorders in athletes is not well defined, research shows it occurs more frequently in sports that emphasize lean-ness.[17,20-23] Sundgot-Borgen[17] examined the prevalence of eating disorders in 522 Norwegian elite female athletes representing 35 different sports. Results of the study showed the prevalence of eating disorders was higher in athletes (18%) than nonathletes (5%), and that eating disorders and the use of patho-genic weight control methods were significantly higher among athletes in aesthetic (34%) and weight-dependent (27%) sports compared to endurance (20%), technical (13%), and team sports (11%) (Figure 7.1). Additionally, the prevalence of eating disorders within sport groups varied significantly. For example, among endurance athletes, middle/long distance runners and cross-country skiers were at greater risk of eating disorders than cyclists, swimmers, and women rowers.

IV. RISK FACTORS FOR EATING DISORDERS

Many sociocultural, familial, and psychological factors have been impli-cated in the development of eating disorders. Some individuals with anorexia nervosa or bulimia nervosa have easily identifiable signs and others do not.

Females are at greater risk because society places greater demands on women to achieve and maintain an ideal body shape. Studies show that even young girls who are underweight for their height are dieting to combat their fears of being overweight.[24] For many girls, weight and dieting concerns appear as early as the age of 9.[25]

Another factor implicated in the development of eating disorders relates to family dynamics. According to Johnson et al.,[26] there is remarkable consis-tency in the descriptions of families of anorexics, with alcoholism and sexual abuse being prevalent.

According to Lindeman,[27] low self-esteem is a well-known trait of indi-viduals with eating disorders and may be a motivating factor in the develop-ment of anorexia and bulimia. Individuals with eating disorders generally have a history of low self-esteem and difficulty with problem-solving and coping with stress as well as emotional instability and withdrawal from social relationships.[28]

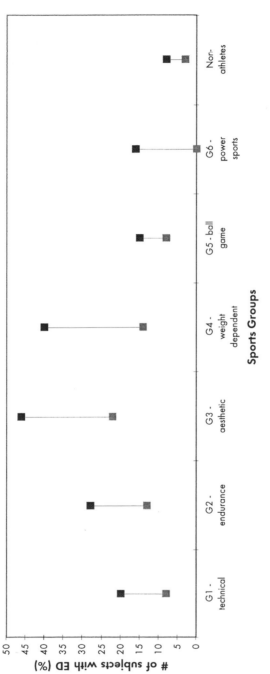
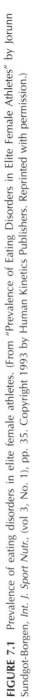

FIGURE 7.1 Prevalence of eating disorders in elite female athletes. (From "Prevalence of Eating Disorders in Elite Female Athletes" by Jorunn Sundgot-Borgen, *Int. J. Sport Nutr.*, (vol 3, No. 1), pp. 35. Copyright 1993 by Human Kinetics Publishers. Reprinted with permission.)

A. DIFFERENCES BETWEEN ATHLETES AND NONATHLETES

The close relationship between body image and athletic performance makes athletes especially vulnerable to an over-emphasis with weight. Although sports that accentuate leanness place athletes at greater risk for developing eating disorders, it is important to recognize that eating disorders occur in athletes in all sports. In a study by Taub and Blinde,[29] sport-by-sport comparisons between track, volleyball, basketball, and softball revealed that softball players scored highest on five of the eight EDI subscales and three of four pathogenic weight control behaviors.

Many factors can account for an athlete's predisposition for eating disorders, including personality characteristics, pressure from coaches and parents to reduce body size for competition, and personality characteristics of athletes. One study[29] has shown that athletes were more likely to be perfectionists and engage in uncontrollable eating behaviors than nonathletes. In another survey,[30] athletes scored higher on bulimia, body dissatisfaction, perfectionism, and drive for thinness subscales than nonathletes.

Williamson et al.[31] used a specific formula to determine risk factors for the development of eating disorder symptoms in female athletes. Researchers tested 98 female college athletes using questionnaires designed to measure (1) social influences for thinness, (2) sports competition anxiety, (3) athletic achievement, and (4) concern with body size and shape. Figure 7.2 presents the psychological model that was tested in their study. Results indicated that pressure from coaches and peers to be thin, combined with anxiety about athletic performance and negative self appraisal of athletic achievement were factors associated with concerns about body size and shape.

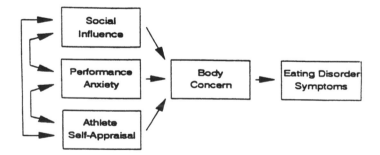

FIGURE 7.2 Psychosocial model tested by Williamson et al. From Williamson, D. A. et al., Structural equation modeling of risk factor for the development of eating disorder symptoms in female athletes, *Int. J. Eat. Disorders,* 17, 392, 1995. Reprinted with permission of John Wiley & Sons, Inc.

Athletes who have developed eating disorders often refer to traumatic experiences with weigh-ins and/or comments from a coach or teammates about body weight. Rosen and Hough[21] reported that 75% of the gymnasts who were told by their coaches that they were too heavy resorted to dangerous weight control measures to lose weight. According to Zucker et al.,[32] young athletes may need only one or two suggestions about reducing body fat before they attempt pathogenic eating behaviors.

Other risk factors that are known to trigger eating disorders are dieting at an early age, frequent weight fluctuations, a sudden increase in training volume, and emotional circumstances such as injury or loss of a coach.[33]

While athletics do not cause an eating disorder, sports-related pressures, high expectations, and comments from coaches about weight and performance can set the stage for development of an eating disorder.

1. Warning Signs

According to Grandjean et al.,[34] there is a distinct difference between being thin and having anorexia, and between vomiting to reach a desired weight and having bulimia. Preoccupations with weight and dieting do not automatically signal an eating disorder. Some athletes may exhibit concerns about body image and take part in anorexic-like behaviors during training but resume normal eating habits and gain weight after the season is over.[35] However, an assessment is warranted if the athlete displays the following warning signs.[36]

Warning Signs for Anorexia Nervosa
- Dramatic loss in weight
- Preoccupation with food, calories, and weight
- Wearing baggy or layered clothing
- Mood swings
- Avoiding food-related social activities

Warning Signs for Bulimia Nervosa
- Noticeable weight loss or gain
- Excessive concern about weight
- Visits to the bathroom following meals
- Depression
- Strict dieting followed by binges
- Increasing criticism of one's body

According to Squire,[37] an important clue to the presence of an eating disorder may be the athlete's response to injury. Many athletes use extreme exercise as a means of controlling weight and become very anxious when an injury prevents them from participating in their regular exercise regimens.[37,38]

V. EFFECTS OF EATING DISORDERS ON HEALTH AND PERFORMANCE

The general medical signs and symptoms of anorexia nervosa and bulimia nervosa have been described and discussed at length elsewhere.[39] This section will briefly review some of the nutrition and performance-related issues affecting athletes with eating disorders.

Athletes with eating disorders typically consume diets low in energy and essential vitamins and minerals. In one of the few studies to assess the nutrient intake of female athletes with eating disorders, Sundgot-Borgen[40] reported that mean carbohydrate intakes were significantly lower than the 8 to 10 g/kg bw/d recommended for optimum performance.[41] The anorexics averaged 1.7 g/kg bw/d with a range of 1.0 to 2.3 g/kg. Low intakes of several nutrients, especially calcium, vitamin D, and iron, were also reported.

Restrictive eating patterns range from poor nutrition to voluntary starvation coupled with extreme exercise regimens.[42] Many athletes cautiously watch the amount of fat they eat, striving for intakes less than 10% of total calories. Dairy foods and high-protein foods such as red meat are often omitted from the diet.[43] Furthermore, as indicated by Sundgot-Borgen,[40] athletes with eating disorders frequently have low carbohydrate intakes which can deplete muscle glycogen stores and reduce endurance capacity.

Prolonged energy restriction and restrictive eating behaviors can lead to serious medical complications such as amenorrhea. As previously stated, decreased estrogen levels associated with amenorrhea can result in decreased bone mineral density and risk for premature osteoporosis. Eating disorders, amenorrhea, and osteoporosis have been the focus of the Female Athlete Triad.[44] Presently, efforts are underway to establish programs for the prevention and treatment of these three disorders in athletes.[45]

VI. EVALUATION AND TREATMENT

While coaches, trainers, sports nutritionists, and parents can identify symptoms that may indicate risk, a diagnosis can only be made by a physician or professional who specializes in eating disorders. The complex multifaceted nature of anorexia and bulimia suggests that an interdisciplinary team consisting of a physician, psychologist, and nutritionist is the best approach to treatment.[46] The physician monitors the athlete's medical condition, the psychologist focuses on family and peer issues as well as body image and eating disordered behaviors, and the nutritionist addresses diet and weight issues, restrictive eating patterns, and co-facilitates body image group therapy.[34]

The members of the team need to work closely together so that messages the athlete receives are consistent. The management team should also have some understanding of the sport environment. For many athletes, their sport is their whole life.[39] Maintaining a scholarship or winning a gold medal may be pursued at any cost.

One of the first issues likely to occur in treating an athlete with an eating disorder is whether or not the athlete should continue to train and compete. According to Harris,[47] the decision should be based on the risk of injury or significant health problems to the athlete. Short-term restrictive eating behaviors or compulsive exercise may not be severe enough to cause serious health risk to the athlete. On the other hand, prolonged starvation, laxative abuse, and self-induced vomiting places the athlete at great health risks and can have a devastating impact on performance.[12] Nattiv[47] believes if the athlete is not willing to comply with treatment, she should not be allowed to stay on the team.

When counseling the athlete with an eating disorder, remember that each athlete's recovery process is unique and treatment plans and goals should be individualized.[46] Weight gain is a priority because many of the existing symptoms of an eating disorder are secondary to starvation.[34] A weight gain of 0.5 kg (1 lb) per week is advised until the athlete achieves her goal weight.[48]

Case studies illustrate the intense emotional anxiety that eating disordered athletes have about food and the fear of getting fat during the first few weeks of treatment.[38,39,48] Visualization techniques, food diaries, and journals are tools often used to help patients verbalize their feelings related to food.[48] The goal is to reverse the athlete's distorted thinking about food, weight, and body image while promoting self esteem and positive feelings about body size.

VII. PREVENTION

Physicians, trainers, coaches, and athletes should be informed about eating disorders and what to do if a problem is suspected. Early detection and intervention are important to the athlete's health and performance. The preparticipation exam provides an opportunity to screen for disordered eating behaviors. Female athletes should be questioned about weight and performance goals. If the athlete displays any warning signs of a possible eating disorder, nutrition counseling should be provided. Questionnaires should be considered merely a screening instrument for further clinical evaluation because data shows that many athletes underreport weight control behaviors.[17]

REFERENCES

1. Pipher, M., *Reviving Ophelia: Saving the Selves of Adolescent Girls*, Grosset Putnam Book, New York, 1994.
2. Stephens, D. L., Hill, R. P., and Hanson, C., The beauty myth and female consumers: the controversial role of advertising, *J. Consumer Affairs*, 28, 137, 1994.
3. Moore, D. C., Body image and eating behavior in adolescent girls, *A.J.D.C.*, 142, 1114, 1988.
4. Werblow, J. A., Fox, H. M., and Henneman, A., Nutritional knowledge, attitudes, and food patterns of women athletes, *J. Am. Diet. Assoc.*, 73, 242, 1978.
5. Parr, R. B., Porter, M. A., and Hodgson, S. C., Nutrition knowledge and practices of coaches, trainers, and athletes, *Phys. Sportsmed.*, 12, 127, 1984.
6. Perron, M. and Endres, J., Knowledge, attitudes, and dietary practices of female athletes, *J. Am. Diet. Assoc.*, 85, 573, 1985.
7. Welch, P. K., Zager, K. A., Endres, J., and Poon, S. W., Nutrition education, body composition, and dietary intake of female college athletes, *Phys. Sportsmed.*, 15, 63, 1987.

8. Dummer, G. M., Rosen, L. W., Heusner, W. W., Roberts, P. J., and Counsilman, J. E., Pathogenic weight-control behaviors of young competitive swimmers, *Phys. Sportsmed.*, 15, 75, 1987.

9. Davis, C. and Cowles, M., A comparison of weight and diet concerns and personality factors among female athletes and non-athletes, *J. Psychoso. Res.*, 33, 527, 1989.

10. American Psychiatric Association, *Diagnostic and Statistical Manual of Mental Disorders*, 4th ed., Washington D. C., American Psychiatric Association, 1994, 539.

11. Sullivan, P. F., Mortality in anorexia nervosa, *Am. J. Psychiatry*, 152, 1073, 1995.

12. Omaha World-Herald, August 15, 1994.

13. Beals, K. A. and Manore, M. M., The prevalence and consequences of subclinical eating disorders in female athletes, *Int. J. Sport Nutr.*, 4, 175, 1994.

14. Sundgot-Borgen, J., Eating disorders in female athletes, *Sports Med.*, 17, 176, 1994.

15. Pugliese, M. T., Lifshitz, F., Grad, G., Fort, P., and Marks-Katz, M., Fear of obesity: A cause of short stature and delayed puberty, *N. Engl. J. Med.*, 309, 513, 1983.

16. Smith, N. J., Excessive weight loss and food aversion in athletes simulating anorexia nervosa, *Pediatrics*, 66, 139, 1980.

17. Sundgot-Borgen, J., Prevalence of eating disorders in elite female athletes, *Int. J. Sport Nutr.*, 3, 29, 1993.

18. Garner, D. M. and Garfinkel, P. E., The eating attitudes test: an index of the symptoms of anorexia nervosa, *Psych. Med.*, 9, 273, 1979.

19. Garner, D. M., Olmstead, M. P., and Polivy, J., Development and validation of a multidimensional eating disorder inventory for anorexia nervosa and bulimia, *Int. J. Eating Disorders*, 2, 15, 1983.

20. O'Connor, P. J., Lewis, R. D., and Kirchner, E. M., Eating disorder symptoms in female college gymnasts, *Med. Sci. Sports Exerc.*, 27, 550, 1994.

21. Rosen, L. W., McKeag, D. B., Hough, D. O., and Curley, V., Pathogenic weight control behavior in female athletes, *Phys. Sportsmed.*, 14, 79, 1986.

22. Rucinski, A., Relationship of body image and dietary intake of competitive ice skaters, *J. Am. Diet. Assoc.*, 89, 98, 1989.

23. Steen, S. N. and McKinney, S., Nutrition assessment of college wrestlers, *Phys. Sportsmed.*, 14, 100, 1986.

24. Koff, E. and Rierdan, J., Perceptions of weight and attitudes toward eating in early adolescent girls, *J. Adoles. Health*, 12, 307, 1991.

25. Mellin, L. M., Irwin, C. E., and Scully, S., Prevalence of disordered eating in girls: a survey of middle-class children, *J. Am. Diet. Assoc.*, 92, 851, 1992.

26. Johnson, C. L., Sansone, R. A., and Chewning, M., Good reasons why young women would develop anorexia nervosa: the adaptive context, *Pediatric Ann.*, 21, 731, 1992.

27. Lindeman, A. K., Self-esteem: its application to eating disorders and athletes, *Int. J. Sport Nutr.*, 4, 237, 1994.

28. Mallick, M. J., Whipple, T. W., and Huerta, E., Behavioral and psychological traits of weight-conscious teenagers: A comparison of eating-disordered patients and high- and low-risk groups, *Adolescence*, 22, 157, 1987.

29. Taub, D. E. and Blinde, E. M., Eating disorders among adolescent female athletes: Influence of athletic participation and sport team membership, *Adolescence*, 27, 833, 1992.

30. Sundgot-Borgen, J. S. and Corbin, C. B., Eating disorders among female athletes, *Phys. Sportsmed.*, 15, 89, 1987.

31. Williamson, D. A., Netemeyer, R. G., Jackman, L. P., Anderson, D. A., Funsch, C. L., and Rabalais, J. Y., Structural equation modeling of risk factors for the development of eating disorder symptoms in female athletes, *Int. J. Eating Disorders*, 17, 387, 1995.

32. Zucker, P., Avener, J., Bayder, S., Brotman, A., Moore, K., and Zimmerman, J., Eating disorders in young athletes, *Phys. Sportsmed.*, 13, 88, 1985.

33. Sundgot-Borgen, J., Risk and trigger factors for the development of eating disorders in female elite athletes, *Med. Sci. Sports Exerc.*, 26, 414, 1994.

34. Grandjean, A. C., Woscyna, G. R, and Ruud, J. S., Eating disorders in athletes, In *Office Sports Medicine*, Mellion, M. B., (Ed.), 2nd ed., Hanley & Belfus, Philadelphia, 1996, 113.
35. Leon, G. R., Eating disorders in female athletes, *Sports Med.*, 12, 219, 1991.
36. Wilmore, J. H., Eating and weight disorders in the female athlete, *Int. J. Sport Nutr.*, 1, 104, 1991.
37. Squire, D. L., Eating disorders, In *Sports Medicine Secrets*, Mellion, M. B., (Ed.)., Hanley & Belfus, Inc., Philadelphia, 1994, 136.
38. Clark, N., How to help the athlete with bulimia: practical tips and a case study, *Int. J. Sport Nutr.*, 3, 450, 1993.
39. Thompson, R. A. and Sherman, R. T., *Helping Athletes with Eating Disorders*, Human Kinetic Publishers, Champaign, 1993.
40. Sundgot-Borgen, J., Nutrient intake of female elite athletes suffering from eating disorders, *Int. J. Sport Nutr.*, 3, 431, 1993.
41. Sherman, W. M. and Wimer, G. S., Insufficient dietary carbohydrate during training: Does it impair performance? *Int. J. Sport Nutr.*, 1, 28, 1991.
42. Johnson, M. D., Disordered eating in active and athletic women, *Clin. Sports Med.*, 13, 355, 1994.
43. Frusztajer, N. T., Dhuper, S., Warren, M. P., Brooks-Gunn, J., and Fox, R. P., Nutrition and the incidence of stress fractures in ballet dancers, *Am. J. Clin. Nutr.*, 51, 779, 1990.
44. Yeager, K. K., Agostini, R., Nattiv, A., and Drinkwater, B., The female athlete triad: disordered eating, amenorrhea, osteoporosis, *Med. Sci. Sports Exerc.*, 25, 775, 1993.
45. Skolnick, A. A., "Female athlete triad" risk for women, *J. Am. Med. Assoc.*, 270, 921, 1993.
46. Position of the American Dietetic Association: Nutrition intervention in the treatment of anorexia nervosa, bulimia nervosa, and binge eating, *J. Am. Diet. Assoc.*, 94, 902, 1995.
47. Harris, S. S. and Nattiv, A., Controversies in Sports Medicine: should women with eating disorders be allowed to participate in athletics? *Sports Medicine Digest*, 17, 1, 1995.
48. Clark, N., Counseling the athlete with an eating disorder: A case study, *J. Am. Diet. Assoc.*, 94, 656, 1994.